Medical & Diagnostic Bacteriology:

A Guide in Resources Constrained Laboratories

I0505084

Vitus Silago
(Health Laboratory Scientist)

i

PREFACE and INTRODUCTION

In low and middle income countries (LMICs), the emerging threat of antimicrobial resistant bacteria causing diseases is a major concern. LMICs face many challenges when implementing laboratory medicine, given the scarcity of diagnostic bacteriology laboratories and availability of limited options of effective antibiotic therapy for resistant pathogens. Consequently increasing morbidity and mortality rates among patients especially in intensive care units (ICUs). Further, limiting the availability of antimicrobial resistance data from LMICs.

Medical Bacteriology is defined as the study of diseases causing bacteria. It covers host-parasite interactions including host defense mechanisms and bacterial virulence factors, a critical step in understanding of bacterial pathogenicity.

Diagnostic Bacteriology is the study of isolation and identification of diseases causing bacteria. Different culture media, depending on the purpose, are used for the isolation of diseases causing bacteria from clinical specimens (e.g., blood, urine and pus). The isolated bacteria are then speciated to possible Genera and/or species by biochemical identification tests. Further, isolates (bacteria) are subjected to in vitro antibiotic susceptibility testing to determine their susceptibility patterns towards different antibiotic agents for the purpose of guiding rational antibiotic therapy.

All diagnostic procedures in Bacteriology Laboratories are centered to quality assurances which ensure the reproducibility and reliability of the produced results. In all stages, quality check should be maintained and documented in accordance to local and international laboratory standards. Moreover, results should be reported within turn-around-time (TAT) for timely initiation of rational antibiotic therapy.

ACKNOWLEDGEMENTS

I am grateful to express my deepest gratitude to the most High God, for His love, mercy and grace in my life.

First I would like to extend my sincerely thanks to my lovely wife: Conjester V. Silago; daughter: Ivanna V. Silago; and son: Isaac V. Silago for their love, understanding and support for the entire period of time I was busy preparing this work.

Second, I would like to thank all members of the Microbiology and Immunology department, Weill Bugando School of Medicine of the Catholic University of Health and Allied Sciences, Bugando (Mwanza, Tanzania) for technical and academic supports they provided me.

Lastly, my special thanks go to Mr. Adam Absalom Mwakyoma (Medical Laboratory Scientist) and Mr. Lukas Michael Sumani (Medical Laboratory Scientist) for their technical support they provided during making of this piece of work.

Table of Contents

CHAPTER ONE

Introduction to bacteria cell: structure, genetic and metabolism

Anatomical structure of bacteria cell

Cell is defined as the smallest unit of life. Basically there are two types of cells, prokaryotic and eukaryotic [1]. Prokaryotic cell is the type of cell which does not contain true nucleus (lack true defined membrane bound nucleus know as nucleoid or nuclear body), mitochondria (or simple chromosome) and true defined membrane bound organelles [1, 2]. Bacteria are the typical example of prokaryotic cell. Eukaryotic cell is the type of cell which contains true nucleus (membrane bound nucleus) and membrane bound organelles [3].

Bacteria cell as typical prokaryotic cell it contains both deoxyribonucleic acid (DNA) and ribonucleic acid (RNA) which replicates by binary fission [1]. Almost all bacteria cells are containing rigid cell walls [2]. Bacteria cell can grow in vitro on artificial culture media in the laboratory. Also, bacteria cells are sensitive to one or more antibiotic agents however there are some strains of bacteria cells possess mechanisms for antibiotics resistance [2, 3].

Structure of bacteria cell

Basically, bacteria cell contains three major components namely cell envelop: cell wall and cell membrane; cellular elements enclosed within cell envelope: ribosomes, nuclear apparatus, mesosomes and other cytoplasmic granules; and cellular elements outside cell envelop: flagella, glycocalyx and pili [3].

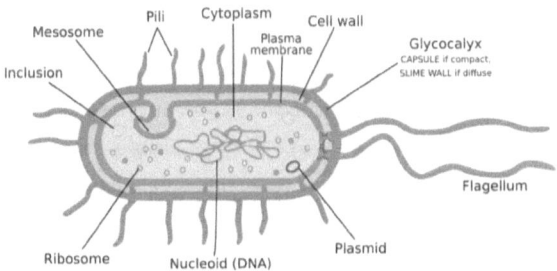

Figure 1: Anatomical structure of bacteria cell (Source: wpclipart [4])

Cell envelope

Cell envelope includes cell wall and cell membrane. Cell wall is a multi-layered structure of thickness between 0.15 and 0.5 μm which consist of about 20% of the total dry weight of the bacteria cell. Thickness of cell wall varies widely between young and rapidly growing (containing thin cell wall) and old and slowly dividing (containing thick cell wall) bacteria cells. Generally bacterial cell wall is structured by N-acetyl muramic acid and N-acetyl Glucosamine back bones cross linked with peptide chain and penta-glycine bridges. However, some variations exist between cell walls of Gram-negative and Gram-positive bacteria. The cell walls of Gram-negative bacteria are mainly composed of phospholipid, lipoprotein, lipopolysaccharide and thin peptidoglycan layer. The cell walls of Gram-positive bacteria is mainly composed of teichoic acid and thick layer of peptidoglycan [3]. This difference of main composition between Gram-positive and Gram-negative bacteria (especially the thickness of peptidoglycan layers) easies their differentiation by Gram stain dyes [2].

The general function of bacterial cell wall include: provides defined shape to the bacterium, protects cytoplasmic contents from external environment, provide rigidity to the organism, provides Gram staining differentiation characteristics between Gram-negative and Gram-positive bacteria, contains receptor sites for bacteriophages and complements immune system, contains toxic components to destroy host cells and tissues, site of action of host's antibody and antibiotics (e.g., cell wall acting antibiotics i.e., beta-lactams) [2, 3].

Sometimes bacteria cells are lacking or containing defective cell walls. There are three types of such kinds of bacteria: spheroplast, protoplast and L-form bacteria. Spheroplast bacteria are Gram-negative bacteria containing non-functional cell wall materials which make it to be very fragile osmotically. They are grown in the presence of penicillin antibiotic. Protoplast bacteria are Gram-positive bacteria which is completely lacking cell wall. They are grown in the presence of lysozyme in hypertonic solution containing medium. L-form bacteria they may exist naturally or produced in vivo when the host is exposed to penicillin antibiotics [3].

Cell membrane sometimes known as cytoplasmic membrane, it is a trilaminar membrane which accounts for 30% of the total dry weight of the bacteria cell. Structurally, it composed of higher protein (about 60%) than carbohydrate (about 15%) and lipids (about 25%). Functionally, cell

2

membrane regulates the transportation of nutrient and waste product across the two cellular environments (outside and inside), captures ATP energy, synthesize materials for cell wall, facilitates DNA replication, and it accommodates the electron transport system [3].

Cellular elements enclosed within cell envelope

Bacterial cellular elements within cell envelop include ribosomes, polyamines, mesosomes, nuclear apparatus and cytoplasmic granules. Ribosomes, this 70S monomer containing two subunits (50S and 30S), it composed of 70% RNA and 30% proteins. Ribosome is the main site of protein synthesis in the bacteria cell. Polyamines exist in three types namely spermine, spermidine and putrescin. In association with ribosomes, cell membrane and DNA, polyamines acts as mutagenic, resist the lysis of protoplast and prevents the degradation of 70S ribosome into its subunits (50S and 30S). Mesosome is an outgrowth (invagination) of cytoplasmic membrane in bacterial cytoplasm which is involved in segregation of bacterial DNA during binary fission. The mesosomes are more common among Gram-positive bacteria than Gram-negative bacteria [2]. Nuclear apparatus, it is called so because it lacks nuclear membrane, mitotic apparatus and discrete chromosome. This is also known as bacterial genome or core genome which consist of circular and double stranded DNA. However, sometimes bacteria may harbor extra chromosomal genetic materials which are acquired via conjugation, transformation or transduction [1]. They have nothing to do with normal functioning of the bacteria cell but they may add some beneficial traits to bacteria for example resistance to antibiotics and virulence factors. Therefore they provide bacteria cell with additional survival adaptations. Cytoplasmic granules are also known as vacuoles, they function as food reserves in bacteria cell.

Cellular elements outside the cell envelop

Outside bacterial cell envelop, there is glycocalyx, pilus and flagellum. Glycocalyx this includes capsule and slime layer. They are both layers of gel but capsule adheres firmly while slime adheres weakly on cell envelop. All bacteria contains at least a thin layer of slime however not all bacteria are containing capsules. Polysaccharides and protein are the major components of capsule. Generally, capsules are antigenic and virulent structure among other bacteria (e.g., capsule in hypervirulent *Klebsiella pneumoniae*), protects bacteria cell from phagocytic host cells, and are detected by quelling phenomenon. Also, most capsulated bacteria cells are non-motile.

Flagellum, this organ consists of three parts which are filament, hook and basal body. The basal body and hook are implanted in the cell surface but the filament is free on the surface [2]. Flagellum is richly made by protein known as flagellin [2]. Flagellum facilitates motility or swimming (propeller-like-action) of bacteria which may be detected as hanging drop (presumptive diagnosis of *Vibrio cholera*), swarming phenomenon on the surface of solid media (*Proteus* species) and turbidity motility in semi-solid media e.g., sulfur-indole-motility agar (*Escherichia coli*) [2]. The movement of basal body which drives the propeller-like-action movement of the entire flagellum is driven by proton motive force rather than ATP directly [2]. Flagellum is an antigen among motile bacteria which is known as H (Hauch) antigen [2].

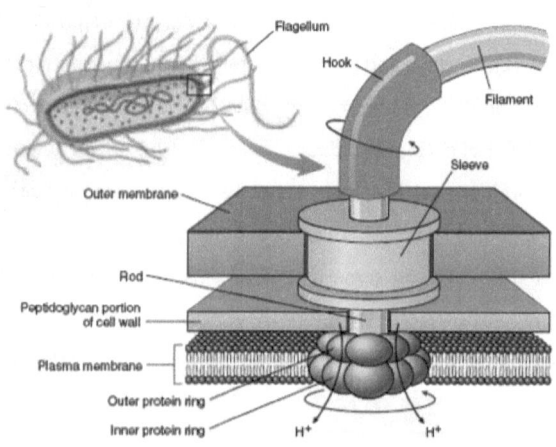

Figure 2: The structure of flagellum (Source: Quora [5])

Flagellar on bacteria cell can be as monotrichous: single flagellum at one pole (e.g., *Vibrio cholera*); lophotrichous: tuft (bunch) of flagella at one pole (e.g., *Bartonella baciliformis*); amphitrichous: single flagellum at both poles (e.g., *Spirillum serpens*); peritrichous: flagella all over bacteria cell (e.g., *Escherichia coli*); and amphilophotrichous: tuft (bunch) of flagella at both poles. Bacteria with no flagellum are known as atrichous and axial filament like-flagella used for motility are known as endoflagella [2].

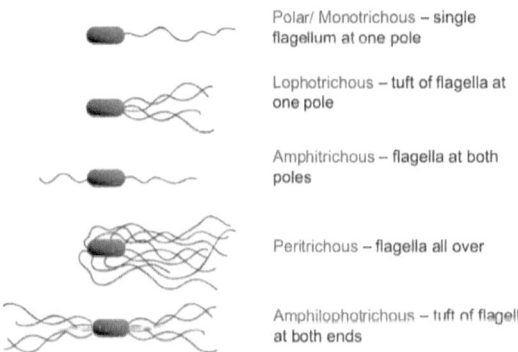

Figure 3: Arrangement of flagella on bacteria cell (Source: Rai University [6])

Pilus (plural pili) also known as fimbriae is hair-like structure which is composed of protein known as pilin [2]. Pili are mainly found in most of Gram-negative bacteria [2]. Based on their function on bacteria cell, there are two types of pili which are common pili (very short) for adherence and sex pili (very long but not as long as flagellum) for conjugation a process which facilitate transfer of mobile genetic element between bacteria cells including plasmid [2]. Sex pili can be differentiated from common pili by their affinity towards male-specific bacteriophages [2].

Bacteria genetics

Genetics is defined as the study of inheritance in organisms from one generation to the next generation. In bacteria, DNA encodes for all traits inheritance from one bacteria cell to the next bacteria cell after binary fission. Bacteria cytoplasm consists of core genome (also known as chromosomal DNA) and other additional (optional) replicons (genomes), either plasmid and/or bacteriophage [2, 3].

Bacteria core genome is circular, double stranded DNA of the size between 0.4×10^9 and 8.6×10^9 Daltons (Da). Bacteria chromosomal DNA is attached to bacterial cell membrane. The smallest chromosomal DNA is contained in obligate parasitic bacteria (i.e., *Mycoplasma*) and the largest core genome is contained in complex differentiating bacteria (i.e., *Myxococcus*).

5

Generally, the chromosomal DNA contributes only about 2-3% to the total bacteria dry weight. Also, in comparison to human chromosomal DNA, bacteria compares to 0.1% only. Replication of chromosomal DNA of bacteria is semi-conservative, each strand of the original DNA during replication it forms its complimentary strand resulting into two chromosomal DNA of which each is containing one original strand of the previous DNA. Then, mother cell is remained with one double stranded DNA and daughter cell receives another double stranded DNA [2, 3].

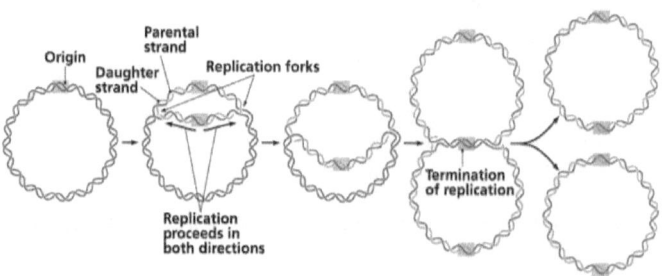

Figure 4: Replication of bacteria chromosomal DNA (Source: Pearson Education Inc., 2006).

Plasmids are discrete extra-chromosomal genetic elements (in bacteria cell) which are supercoiled, circular and double stranded DNA. In some few bacteria exists linear plasmids (e.g., *Streptomyces* and *Borrelia* species). Normally, the size of plasmid ranges from five to hundreds kilobase pairs however plasmids of up to 2Mbp exists I some bacteria. Plasmid of sizes less than 7.5 kbp are normally not conjugative. Plasmids are self-replicating, multiplies independent of the host cell. Therefore, multiple copies of the same plasmid may be present in one bacteria however different plasmids may also be present in one bacteria. Mainly there are three types of plasmid: F (fertility) plasmid or F factor, promotes the transfer of chromosomal DNA from mother cell to daughter cell by recombining itself with chromosomal DNA; R plasmid or R factor, they determines resistance to antibiotics by carrying antibiotics resistance encoding genes; and Col plasmid or Col factor they are carrying extracellular toxin encoding genes [3].

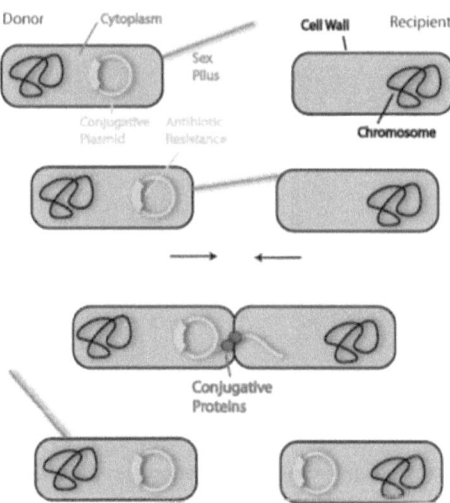

Figure 5: Transfer of plasmid between donor and recipient bacteria cell by conjugation process (Source: Pinterest by Katrina Howarth)

Bacteriophages are bacteria viruses also known as phages. They are replicating in bacteria cells as obligate intracellular parasites. Outside bacteria cell, phage replication is not possible. Phages contain nucleic acid (either single or double stranded DNA or RNA, but not both) incased in a protein protective capsid. Phage nucleic acid varies in size from 2 to 200 kbp. Phage genome codes for own-replication, synthesis of capsid and non-structural protein responsible for progenies (phage daughters) assembly. During bacterial infection, only phage nucleic acid is entering bacteria cell, its capsid remains at the cell surface. In bacteria cell, phage replicates into many new copies which after their assembly may leave or stay in the bacteria cytoplasm. The release of phage from bacteria cell results into death of the host cell by lysis. Therefore, there are two types of phages, virulent and temperate. Virulent phages leave host cell after assembly resulting to cell lysis. Temperate phages are of two types, lytic phage and lysogenic phage. Lytic phages are similar to virulent phages. Lysogenic phages are latent, living with bacteria cell and not causing lysis [2].

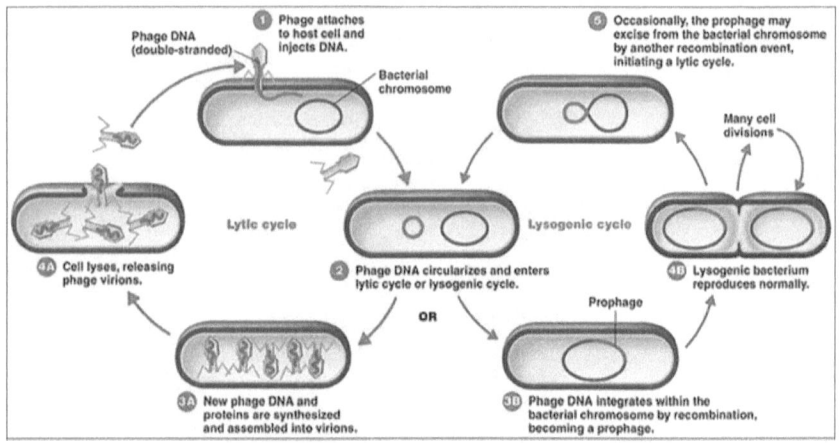

Figure 6: The lytic and lysogenic cycles of bacteriophage (Source: eNotes Editorial [7])

Bacteriophages: antibacterial therapy against multidrug resistant bacteria

The upsurge of antibiotic resistant bacteria, a global concern, has awakened the therapy concept of bacteriophage. Because bacteriophage infects bacteria specifically. Phage infecting *Staphylococcus aureus* cannot infect *Escherichia coli* or any other cell in bacterial host's body (i.e., human cells) [8]. Phages are self-regulating at the site of infection with no single negative side effect such as toxicity [8]. Once infectious bacteria have been killed, phages decay spontaneously. Also, phage availability is not an issue, because they are ubiquitous in nature and all the time bacteria co-evolve with their specific phages. There are commercially available phages however some laboratories can prepare their own phages for therapy [9].

Therefore, phages provide hope of modern medicine as treatment therapy for multidrug resistant bacteria. Once they binds to their specific receptors on bacteria cell, they inject their nucleic acid, replicates to multiple copies which assembles into capsid and upon leaving host cell (bacteria) they are killing it by lysis. However not all phages qualifies as phage therapy, its only well characterized and highly purified obligate lytic phages (virulent phages). Phage therapy cannot replace antibiotic therapy but can be applied simultaneously as they work synergistically [8].

Phage therapy is reported to provide effective lytic activity of 84-100% against multidrug resistant bacteria, methicillin resistant *Staphylococcus aureus* (MRSA) and extended spectrum beta-lactamase (ESBL) producing *Enterobacteriaceae* [9]. One patient of 15 years with cystic fibrosis and disseminated drug resistant *Mycobacterium abscessus* was successful healed after intravenous therapy with three phage cocktail which efficiently killed infectious bacteria [10].

Bacterial metabolism

Bacterial metabolism is defined as biochemical reactions taking place in within bacteria cell. In bacteria, metabolism focuses on dissimilation reactions which functions to generate energy and assimilation reactions in which bacteria uptake and utilizes organic and inorganic compounds for their growth and maintenance of cellular homeostasis. The two reactions are catalyzed by enzymatic controlled system and the overall end-product is the self-replication of the bacteria cell.

From physiology of bacteria nutrition or metabolic aspects, there are three types of bacteria: heterotrophs, autotrophs and phototrophs. Heterotrophic bacteria obtain their energy from oxidation of organic compounds (mostly pathogenic bacteria) of carbohydrate (mainly glucose), protein and lipids. The main product of these oxidative reactions of organic compounds is energy in form of ATP, however other by-products are used as precursor molecules for assimilation reactions. Phototrophic bacteria reduce CO_2 to carbohydrate (mostly glucose). They synthesize their own intracellular glucose for own biosynthesis or energy production. Examples of phototrophic bacteria are *Heliobacterium chlorum* and *Halobacterium salinarium*. Autotrophic bacteria are slowly growing bacteria at the expenses of mineral ions (inorganic compounds). They use CO_2 as their source of carbon and nitrogen containing compounds (N_2, NH_3 or NO_3^-) as their source of nitrogen. Most autotrophic bacteria are not easily isolated (grown) artificially on culture media containing organic compounds. Other autotrophic bacteria are sulfur (H_2S, S, and S_2O_3) oxidizing (e.g., *Thiobacillus ferrooxidans*) [2].

References

1. Guerrero R, Berlanga M: **The hidden side of the prokaryotic cell: rediscovering the microbial world**. *International Microbiology* 2007, **10**(3):157.
2. Baron S: **Classification--Medical Microbiology**: University of Texas Medical Branch at Galveston; 1996.
3. Tadesse A, Alem M: **Medical Bacteriology**. *University of Gondar* 2006.

4.   Bacteria cell diagram
     [https://www.wpclipart.com/medical/microscopic/bacteria/bacteria_cell_diagram.png.
     html]
5.   Are prokaryotic flagella and eukaryotic flagella different in structure?
     [https://www.quora.com/Are-prokaryotic-flagella-and-eukaryotic-flagella-different-in-
     structure]
6.   Bacteria morphology and classification [https://www.slideshare.net/raiuniversity/bsc-
     micro-i-em-unit-31-bactria]
7.   Compare and contrast the lytic and lysogenic life cycles of a virus
     [https://www.enotes.com/homework-help/compare-contrast-lytic-lysogenic-life-cycles-
     virus-635908]
8.   Rohde C, Wittmann J, Kutter E: **Bacteriophages: A Therapy Concept against Multi-
     Drug–Resistant Bacteria.** *Surgical infections* 2018, **19**(8):737-744.
9.   Kutateladze M, Leshkasheli L, Bolkvadze D, Askilashvili L, Balarjishvili N: **Bacteriophages
     against multidrug resistant bacterial infections.** *International Journal of Infectious
     Diseases* 2016, **53**:46-47.
10. Dedrick RM, Guerrero-Bustamante CA, Garlena RA, Russell DA, Ford K, Harris K, Gilmour
     KC, Soothill J, Jacobs-Sera D, Schooley RT: **Engineered bacteriophages for treatment of
     a patient with a disseminated drug-resistant Mycobacterium abscessus.** *Nature
     medicine* 2019, **25**(5):730.

CHAPTER TWO

An overview to Immunology of bacterial infections

Antibodies (immunoglobulins)

Recently known as specific neutralizing substances or antitoxin (by von Behring and Kitasato) these Y shaped substances are now recognized as antibodies (immunoglobulins). Naturally, they are glycoproteins presnt in serum (and others in body fluids), their production is induced by invasion of antigens (immunogenic substances) of which they reacts and binds specifically to the provoking antigens [1].

Structurally, antibodies are composed of 2 light chains and 2 heavy chains. The light chains are the same throughout different classes of antibodies but the heavy chains differ from one class of antibody to another. This difference provides five different classes (epitopes) of antibodies namely, Immunoglobulin-M, G, A, E and D (IgM, IgG, IgA, IgE and IgD). Moreover, some classes of immunoglobulins are further subdivided into subclasses. Both chains, heavy and light consist of domains with variable and constant sequences. For heavy chains the domains are V_H (variable) and C_H (constant) while for light chains the domains are V_L (variable) and C_L (constant). Also, antibodies divided into Fab region having paratope for antigens binding and fragment crystalizable (Fc) region which is similar among same isotypes [2].

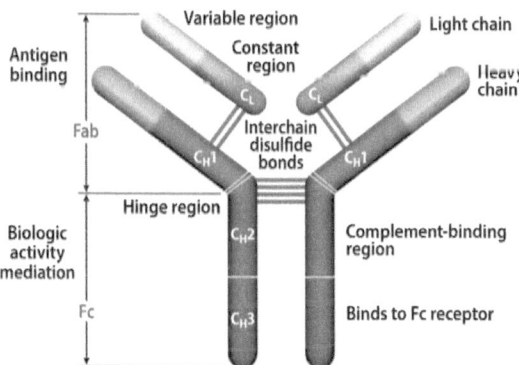

Figure 1: General structure of immunoglobulin (Source: www.myeloma.org)

Types of immunoglobulins

IgM: it is a pentamer molecule containing μ heavy chain. Found intravascularly, it is the first responder (first produced) during immune reaction.

IgG: this second responder containing γ heavy chain has four subclasses; IgG1, IgG2, IgG3 and IgG4. About 75% of serum antibodies is IgG. Also, it can be found in tissues.

IgA: containing α heavy chain, this monomer molecule (in humans) known as secretory immunoglobulin G (sIgG) because it is found in seromucous secretions (colostrum, tears, saliva, mucosal secretions of the gastrointestinal tract, respiratory tract and vagina). It has two subclasses; IgA1 and IgA2.

IgE: this immunoglobulin contains ε heavy chain. Mast cells and basophils contain specific receptors for Fc regions of this immunoglobulin, therefore they are always found on the surfaces of these cells.

IgD: containing δ heavy chain, they are carried by B cells in the serum although very low (<1%).

Antigens (immunogens)

Antigens are substances with the ability to provoke immune response and therefore production of specific antibodies towards provoking substance and no other cells in the host body. This response is not towards the entire provoking substance (antigen) but towards a certain part within it [3]. Simply, it is like "lock and key theory". Consider an antibody as a key and an antigen as a lock. Key enters specifically into a key hole on the lock to open the lock, the same; antibody reacts with just a part of antigen. Mostly, immunoglobulins are produced after exposure to antigens leading to acquired immune system which is divided into cell-mediated and humoral responses.

General function of antibodies

Generally, antibodies functions as neutralizing agents, compliment activators and cell binding and opsonizing substances [4, 5]. Neutralization is by agglutination of antigens through binding of divalent antibody to multivalent antigen to form immune complex (antibody-antigen complex). No antibody can agglutinate an antigen with single epitope. Antibodies (IgM at the C_H3 domain and IgG at the C_H2 domain) binds to the subunit of the first component of complement cascade (C1q) resulting to inflammatory reactions and cell lysis. This is what known as activation of complements system. Cell binding and opsonization is when antibody-antigen complex binds to phagocyte. The binding is between Fc region of the antibody and Fc receptor on the phagocyte. Then, an antigen is phagocytized into phagocyte while antibody is left free for next serve [4].

Antigen recognition

Immune system is supposed to protect host body from potentially pathogenic antigens (microorganism) such as bacteria, viruses, fungi and parasites. But immune system should recognize microbes only and not host's cells. This is achieved through cell-mediated and humoral immunity arms of the acquired immune system. Another type of immune system, innate immune system protects the body from entry of microbes naturally.

Types of immune systems and their roles against invading antigens (bacteria)

All cells of the immune systems originate from either myeloid or lymphoid progenitors in bone marrow. Refer the below figure.

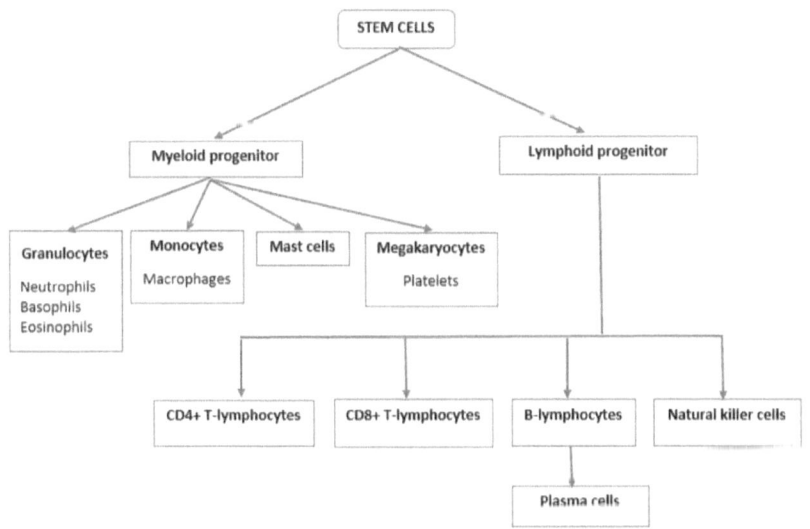

Figure 2: Cells of the immune systems originating from stem cells in bone marrow

Innate immunity

Innate immunity is the type of immune system which healthy individuals are born with. It is non-specific. This type of immunity provides secretions and physical barriers against colonization and invasion of microorganism such as bacteria. This is initial defence mechanisms of the body against microorganisms. This type of immune system recognizes unique structures on bacteria such as lipopolysaccharides, lipoteichoic acid and peptidoglycans. The components of innate immune system are macrophages, Toll like receptors, neutrophils, dendritic cells, epithelial cells and endothelial cells of different mucosal surfaces [6].

Mechanisms of innate immune system against bacteria

Mechanisms of innate immunity to prevent pathogenic bacteria from colonization and invasion includes; surface secretions and physical barriers, humoral defence mechanism, compliment system and cells [7].

Surface secretions and physical barriers

Keratinized skin plays major role in preventing bacteria from accessing into susceptible epidermis cells because most bacteria cannot digest keratin-containing skin. Also, bactericidal and fungicidal fatty acids in sweats and sebaceous secretions provide effective protections against bacteria. In respiratory tract mucosal surface secrets sticky mucus which traps pathogenic bacteria which are then swept together with the trapping mucus by ciliary movement of the cilia (hair-like structures) towards oropharynx where they can be swallowed or spit. Hydrochloric acid (HCL) secreted by stomach kills most of bacteria eaten in contaminated food. Also, bacteria are stopped from colonizing and invading the urinary tract system by flushing action of urine and from eyes by the washing action of tears [7].

Complement system

This system includes numerous serum proteins however in low concentrations but they can destroy cells of Gram-negative bacteria. Usually these serum proteins exist inactively. When activated, its cascade is self-monitored; product of the previous reaction is the catalyst of the next reaction. Two pathways, classical and alternative, are taken to activate complement system but both produces the same physiological effects which are opsonization, activation and lysis (killing) of bacteria [7].

Phagocyte cells

These cells contain digestive enzymes which digests bacteria upon their engulfing. However some bacteria can resist digestion by these cells for example *Mycobacteria* may resist digestion by macrophages.

Humoral defence mechanisms

These microbicidal substances (interferons, lysozymes, acute-phase proteins and basic polypeptides) found in tissues and body fluids produces molecules that destroys bacteria. Basic polypeptides (spermidine, spermine and histone) hydrolyze bacteria cell walls through reacting with acid polysaccharides. Lysozymes (mucolytic enzymes) kill most of Gram-positive bacteria by hydrolyzing their cell walls through splitting of peptidoglycan sugars. Acute-phase proteins, mostly it is C-reactive protein binds phodphorylcholine residues of bacteria cell walls limiting their spreading. Interferons facilitates resistance of humans' cells towards bacterial re-infections [7].

Inflammation

Bacteria produces (or possesses) specific molecules that are recognized by pattern recognition receptors. This recognition triggers the release of cytokines at the site of infection or entry. Tissue damaging bacterial toxins together with these cytokines stimulate inflammatory reactions which increases vascular permeability and vasodilation resulting to accumulation of antibodies, serum protein, complement components, phagocytes, clotting factors and increased blood flow at the site of infection or entry [8, 9]. The effect is catalyzed anaphylatoxins produced by complement components which further the accumulation of fluid and cells at the site. This is the transition from non-specific innate immunity responses towards specific acquired immunity responses.

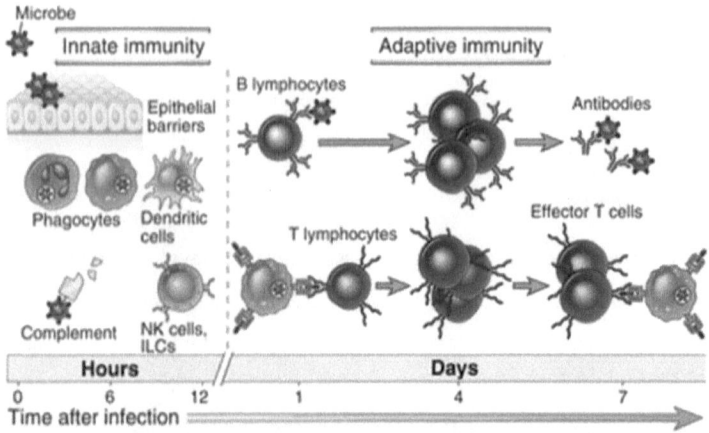

Figure 3: Innate immune system provides non-specific initial defense against microbes. Later on, specific acquired immune system develops after being activated by lymphocytes (Source: Cellular and molecular Immunology, 8th Edition).

Acquired (adaptive) immunity

This specific type of immunity is acquired through exposure to bacteria. To be initiated, this type of immune system requires to be presented with an antigen (bacteria) after its overcoming of the first line of defense (innate immunity). Initiation of specific response of acquired immune system can be in the form of humoral or cell-mediated depending on antigenic nature, route of entry of an antigen and status of the infected host. There are two types of acquired immunity; passive and active. Active acquired immunity is any localized response towards infecting bacteria which is mediated by phagocytes and T-lymphocytes. Passive acquired immunity is introduced to an individual in a form of preformed antibodies such as vaccines [10].

Humoral acquired immunity

Production of antibodies which takes 4 phases (lag, log, plateau and decline) requires an introduction of an antigen. Lag phase is when immune system interacts with an antigen therefore production of antibodies start. During lag phase, antibodies level is too low to be detected. Log phase, this is an exponential rise of produced antibodies and they can be detected. Plateau phase, this is when production and removal of antibodies reach equilibrium. Decline phase, in this phase the clearing of antigen-antibody complexes decrease concentration

16

of antibodies proportionally. However IgA cannot stimulate inflammatory reactions, but it can inhibit bacteria from colonizing mucosal surfaces. Meaning that, any damage to mucosal surfaces provides opportunity of entry for pathogenic bacteria. Most pathogenic bacteria produce exotoxins which penetrates mucosal barriers and results into disease conditions such as cholera, diphtheria and botulism. Both passive acquired (from immunization) and active acquired (from pre-exposure) antibodies can neutralize these toxins by preventing interaction of toxins (most are enzymes in nature) with their substrates [10].

Cell mediated acquired immunity

B cells and T cells promote production of first responding immunoglobulin (IgM) which can switch to secondary responding immunoglobulin (IgG). Then memory cells are produced from antigen-reactive cells. During re-exposure to the same pathogen, memory cells mainly IgG are activated and produced at this time the concentration is ten or more times than before. Furthermore, macrophages are activated by endotoxins on the cell walls of Gram-negative bacteria. Macrophages engulf, kill and remove bacteria, and then the circle start until no bacteria is left. Even extracellular killed bacteria are removed by macrophages. Also, there is a lytic mechanism which does not involve engulfment of bacteria but effector cells (cytotoxic cells) conjugate target cells (bacteria) and cytoplasmic granules containing tumor necrotic factor alpha (TNF-α), interferon-γ, NK cytotoxic factor and TNF-β concentrates at the side of target cell. Upon release of granule contents toward target cell results into target cell death [10].

Introduction to medically important bacteria

Bacteria cell wall and principles of Gram stain

Bacteria are mainly classified into two large groups, Gram-positive and Gram-negative. Classification of bacteria into these groups based on the structure of bacterial cell walls. Bacterial cell walls react different towards two main dyes of the Gram stain test developed by Hans Christian Gram in 1882 and published later in 1884. Gram stain test composed of crystal violet as primary dye, lugol's iodine as mordant, 10% acetone in alcohol (95% ethanol) as decolorizer and safranin or dilute basic carbol fuchsin as secondary dye. Gram stain test is initial test in identifying bacteria and directing the choice of conventional biochemical tests for identifying bacteria to species levels. Thickness of peptidoglycan layer (refer image below) determines bacterial cell wall's reactions towards Gram stain test dyes. In Gram positive bacteria, cell walls are composed with thick peptidoglycan layer while in Gram negative bacteria, cell walls are composed with thin peptidoglycan layer. Thick peptidoglycan layer resists decolonization with Gram stain decolorize therefore retaining primary dye hence bacteria will be seen as bluish or purplish under microscope. These bacteria are known as Gram-positive bacteria. On the other hand, thin peptidoglycan layer loses primary dye upon decolonization with Gram stain decolorizer therefore taking up secondary dye which give bacteria reddish or pinkish color under microscope. These bacteria are known as Gram-negative bacteria. Interpretation of Gram stain test basically considers shape; cocci (spherical-shaped), bacillus (rod-shaped) and spirochetes (spiral shaped), and Gram stain reaction; blue or purple (Gram-positive bacteria) and red or pink (Gram-negative bacteria).

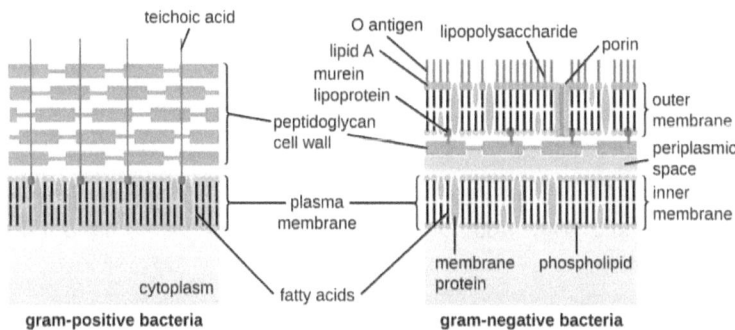

Figure 4: Composition of bacteria cell walls. The difference between Gram-positive and Gram-negative bacteria cell walls (Source: Creative-Biolabs [11])

Gram-positive bacteria
Gram-positive cocci

Cocci (singular coccus) are bacteria with spherical or round shapes however they vary in sizes. Gram-positive cocci bacteria contain multiple genera of medically importance that are *Staphylococci*, *Streptococci*, *Diplococci* and *Enterococci*. They can appear as chains, pairs or clusters as determined by their attachment during cell division. This attachment of one cell to another and their arrangement in general is affected by plane of division. Different arrangements of bacteria cells identify members of some genera. For example, cocci arranged in groups or clusters like a bunch of grapes represents members of *Staphylococci* and cocci arranged in chains like string of beads represents members of *Streptococci* [12].

Staphylococcus

Staphylococcus species are Gram-positive cocci bacteria in the family Staphylococcaceae of the Bacillales order. They are spherical in shape, arranged in groups or cluster like a bunch of grapes. They were first described by Scottish surgeon, Alexander Ogston in 1880 as responsible for pus forming diseases in humans. Two prefixes, staphylo (staphyle in Greek meaning bunch of grapes) and coccus (kokkos in Greek meaning berry or grain) were combined to form the name "Staphylococcus". Generally, *Staphylococcus* bacteria are non motile, non-spore formers, facultative anaerobes, non-capsulated and they are catalase positive. Being positive to catalase, differentiate *Staphylococcus* bacteria from *Streptococcus* bacteria. Recently, there are at least

19

40 species in the genus Staphylococcus of which most of them are harmless and permanent residents of the skin and mucous membranes of humans and some animals [9]. Staphylococci grows on culture media containing up to 10% NaCl (this explains why they can resides on skin) at a temperature ranged between 18^{0}C and 40^{0}C but they grows best at 37^{0}C. Selective mannitol salt (7.5% NaCl) agar can be used to isolate Staphylococci whereby *S. aureus* only can ferment mannitol and gives yellowish colonies that can be differentiated from other Staphylococci.

Staphylococcus aureus

S. aureus are known in implication of number of bacterial infections that can be nosocomial or community acquired. Nosocomial-acquired infections are very common than community-acquired infections. Indwelling devices such as urinary catheters, artificial heart valves, cardiovascular devices and joint prostheses increases the risk of acquisition of nosocomial infections by *S. aureus* [13]. These infections are grouped into pyogenic and toxic mediated infections. Impetigo, bloodstream infections, osteomyelitis, surgical site infections, mastitis, endocarditis, furuncles and boils are pyogenic infections caused by *S. aureus*. Food poisoning, scalded skin syndrome and pemphigus neonatum are grouped as toxin mediated infections caused by *S. aureus* [9]. On sheep blood agar, *S. aureus* produces golden-yellowish colonies with beta hemolysis characteristic.

Pathogenesis of *S. aureus*

For *S. aureus* to cause different human infections it should overcome host defence mechanisms and be able to adhere, invade, survive in or colonize tissues and multiply and damage host tissues. This ability is achieved through different potential virulence factors that are cell surface-associated and extracellular proteins [13].

Adherence

S. aureus produces cell-wall associated adhesins that facilitates recognition and attachment to host's matrix proteins such as fibronectin, collagen and fibrinogen. These adhesins refer to microbial surface components recognizing adhesive matrix molecules (MSCRAMMs). They also produces fibrin-binding protein (fibrinogen) which facilitates attachment to traumatized tissues and blood clots [14].

Overcome of host defence mechanisms

S. aureus produces staphylococcal superantigen-like (SSL) molecules such as SSL3, SSL5 and SSL11 that inhibits neutrophils extravasation and chemotaxis in host body. Through secretion of inhibitory factors, complement activation and phagocytosis of *S. aureus* is blocked. Phagocytosed bacteria inhibits neutrophil-mediated killing by production of inhibitors and enzymes such as adenosine-synthesizing enzyme (AdsA). Moreover, *S. aureus* impairs immune cell functions and cell lysis by expression of β-barrel pore forming toxins (β-PFTs) that binds on specific receptors of immune cells [15]. Furthermore, peptidoglycan layer of most strains is covered with surface protein known as *Staphylococcus* protein A (SpA) which has great affinity towards Fc receptor of Immunoglobulin G (IgG) therefore interfering with opsonization [16].

Damage of host tissues

S. aureus produces wide range of toxins and extracellular enzymes that damage host's tissue they are invading. Some of toxins and extracellular enzymes and their functions are;

Leucocidin; these are exotoxin which disrupt membranes of polymorph-nuclear white blood cells therefore they have lethal effect on these cells.

Enterotoxin; about 65% of *S. aureus* strains produces these superantigen exotoxins which causes gastrointestinal symptoms of staphylococcal food poisoning within 2 to 5 hours after ingestion. There are A-E, G, H, I and J types of enterotoxins which can be produced singly or in combination. These exotoxins are resistant to gastric and duodenal enzymes and they are resistant to boiling (100°C) for 30 minutes. Mainly produced by phage groups III and IV.

Alpha hemolysins (alpha toxins); these chromosomally encoded toxins have hemolysis effect on red blood cells, white blood cells and platelets.

Exfoliatin (epidermolytic toxins); there are two types of epidemolytic toxins; A and B which induces intraepidermal blisters that lead to separation and loss of most of superficial layers of the epidermis resulting to scalded skin syndrome or Ritter disease.

Toxic shock syndrome toxin (TSS); this superantigen toxin was discovered in the early 1980s linked with the use of superabsorbent tampons among women during menstruation. The use of tampons facilitated an overgrowth of *S. aureus* resulting to massive production of TSS. Some species of Streptococci are known to produce toxic shock like (TSL) syndrome toxins specifically group A streptococci (GAS), *S. pyogenes.* These superantigens causes over-activation of cytokines (tumor necrotic-α and interleukin-1) and inflammatory cells by bypassing the normal activation of T cells. These cytokines and inflammatory cells mediate fever, rash, hypotension, tissue injury which results to end-organ failure and shock which is very fatal and life-threatening [17, 18].

Coagulase; this enzyme activates prothrombin nonproteolytically without fVa and fXa cleavage therefore mediates clotting of soluble fibrinogen, plasma and blood [19]. Basically *S. aureus* strains produce one or two types of coagulase; free and/or bound coagulases. Extracellular free coagulase enzyme reacts with prothrombin to mediate coagulation while cell surface coagulase enzyme reacts with α and β of plasma fibrinogen to mediate coagulation. Production of coagulase enzyme by *S. aureus* is significantly used to distinguish *S. aureus* from other Staphylococci species and potential indication that the strain is pathogenic [20, 21].

Staphylococcus saprophyticus

Staphylococcus saprophyticus is coagulase negative *Staphylococci* (CoNs), gamma (no) hemolytic on sheep blood agar, usually implicates in uncomplicated urinary tract infection (UTI) among sexually active females aged between 16 and 25 years. However, can cause complicated infections among immunocompromised and elderly individuals. Furthermore, sometimes they are responsible for epididymitis, prostatitis, urethritis and acute pyelonephritis [22].

Staphylococcus epidermidis

These coagulase negative *Staphylococci* (CoNS) mainly resides on human of which over 85% of human skin normal flora is composed of *S. epidermidis.* They can slowly grow on culture media containing 10% NaCl, sensitive to novobiocin and they are gamma (no) hemolytic on sheep blood agar. Sensitivity to novobiocin differentiates *S. epidermidis* from *Staphylococcus saprophyticus.* Most of them are resistant to multiple antibiotics and associated with healthcare acquired infections such as periodontitis, pericoronitis, acute and chronic pulpitis, angular stomatitis and catheter associated urinary tract infection (CA-UTI). Indwelling urinary catheters, intravenous lines, prosthetic heart valves and shunts increase the risk of acquiring infections by *S. epidermidis* [23].

Streptococcus

Streptococci species are Gram-positive cocci belonging in the family Streptococcaceae under Lactobacillales order. In 1877, Viennese surgeon, Albert Theodor Billroth documented the name by combining two prefixes; strepto (meaning "easily twisted" in Ancient Greek) and coccu (meaning "berry or grain or seed" in Ancient Greek). During cell division, Streptococci take single axis/plane so they grow by forming chains or pairs with twisted or bent appearance. Streptococci are non-motile, non-spore forming, catalase negative (used to differentiate them from Staphylococcus which are catalase positive) and oxidase negative [24]. Three different grouping systems were used to group Streptococci into different groups depending on different similarities and distinct (Table 1) [9].

Table 1: Classification of Streptococci according to type of hemolysis, Lancefield groups and phylogenetic groups

Hemolysis type	Lancefield group	Phylogenetic group	Species
β	A	Pyogenic (pus forming)	S. pyogenes
β	B		S. agalactiae
α	O	Mitis (normal flora of the human oral cavity)	S. pneumoniae
α	O		S. mitis
α	-		S. oralis
α	H		S. sanguinis
α or β	C, G, F	Anginosus (normal flora of the human oral cavity)	S. anginosus
α	-		S. intermedius
-	-	Mutans (colonizes teeth surfaces of human and other animals)	S. sobrinus
-	-		S. mutans
α or none	D	Bovis (normal flora of the colon)	S. bovis

Streptococcus pyogenes

It is also known as group A streptococcus (GAS) because it harbors Lancefield group A antigen. GAS is aerotorelant and extracellular. The name pyogenes come from *pyo* (meaning "pus") and *genes* (from "forming genes"). GAS infections are grouped into non-invasive and invasive streptococcal infections/disease. Pharyngitis, scarlet fever, skin infections such as impetigo and

23

pyoderma are non-invasive streptococcal infections. Streptococcal toxic shock syndrome, necrotizing fasciitis and bacteremia are invasive streptococcal infections. Sometimes, GAS is responsible for rheumatic fever and acute glomerulonephritis which are the results of host immune reactions due to streptococcal infections [25]. *S. pyogenes* are intrinsically resistant to trimethoprim-sulfamethoxazole (SXT) and sensitive to bacitracin, hence these two antibiotic discs are used to distinguish *S. pyogenes* from other beta hemolytic Streptococci such as *S. agalactiae.*

Pathogenesis of *S. pyogenes*

S. pyogenes produces virulence factors which are responsible for adherence, invasion, escaping immunity reactions and damaging of host tissues.

Adhesion; by using surface protein known as F protein, *S. pyogenes* binds to host matrix protein a fibronectin whereby the interaction between the two mediates internalization of *S. pyogenes* into host's cells. M protein and lipoteichoic acid are reported to be involved in adherence to host epithelia cells of the skin and mucous membranes. Attachment to host matrix protein is an initial step of infection by *S. pyogenes* [26].

M protein; are cell surface-exposed protein but anchored in the cytoplasmic membrane responsible for resisting phagocytosis by polymorph-nuclear white blood cells. Antiphagocytic activity of M proteins and its affinity towards some of host's plasma proteins (albumin, IgG, IgA, plasminogen and fibrinogen) are responsible for the ability of *S. pyogenes* to resist phagocytosis [9].

Complement C3b-degrading protease; *S. pyogenes* escapes host immune system by production of this enzyme which cleaves human complements; C3 and C3b which deals to promote opsonization of bacteria. This provide evidence why in some case of invasive infections of *S. pyogenes* there is no neutrophils' infiltration around the bacteria [26].

Glyceraldehyde 3-phosphate dehydrogenase (GAPDH); S. pyogenes produces GAPDH which induces cleavage of host (human) complement C5a, a known chemotaxin which attracts neutrophils to the sites of infections [26].

Streptolysins (SLs); two types, SL-O and SL-S. SL-O activates platelets and endotherial cells resulting to perfusion deficit that ischemically destruct other tissues while cytolysin SL-S is known to promote or induce lysis of red blood cells [27].

Pyrogenic exotoxins; these fatal and fever inducing exotoxins include SPE-A, SPE-B, SPE-C and SPE-G to M. SPE-A is the most toxic "superantigen" exotoxin produced by *S. pyogenes* which is associated with scarlet fever [27]. Generally, these exotoxins cause over-release of cytokines (interleukin 1 & 2, tumor necrotic factor α and interferon γ) which induces inflammation, hypotensive shock and organ failure and final death.

Deoxyribonucleases (streptodornase DNase); they are four enzymes with deoxyribonuclease activity produced by *S. pyogenes* namely A, B, C and D whereby B is the most antigenic. In addition to deoxyribonuclease activities, deoxyribonucleases B and D have ribonuclease activities [28]. These enzymes allow bacteria to escape neutrophil extracellular traps.

Streptococcus pneumoniae

S. pneumoniae is alpha hemolytic, non-motile and non-spore forming Gram-positive cocci that are always found in pairs, was first isolated from saliva by Louis Pasteur in 1881. *S. pneumoniae* asymptomatically colonize respiratory tract, nasal cavity and sinuses of healthy humans. This bacterium is mostly responsible for community acquire pneumonia (CAP) and meningitis definitely among elderly and children. However, it can also cause bronchitis, otitis media, septicemia and meningitis. *S. pneumoniae* are positive (sensitive) to optochin test which is used to distinguish them from other alpha hemolytic Streptococci such as Viridans Streptococci [29, 30].

Pathogenesis of *S. pneumoniae*

Capsule; it is polysaccharide in nature which inhibit deposition of complement and phagocytosis by hindering leukocytes from fixed complement on cell walls hence known as antiphagocytic [31].

Pneumolysin; this intracellular protein belongs the family of thiol-activated toxins which is not secreted by pneumococci but can be released by the influence of autolysin. Pneumolysin stimulates human monocytes to produce inflammatory cytokines (tumor necrotic factor-α and interleukin-1β) which inhibits movement of cilia on human respiratory epithelial cells therefore decreasing bactericidal activities, neutrophil chemotaxis, lymphocytes proliferation and synthesis of antibodies [31].

Autolysin; its effects are mediated by the release of pneumolysin. It is responsible for autolysis (lysis) of the bacteria by breaking of peptide cross-linking of peptidoglycan in bacteria cell walls [31].

Viridans streptococci

Viridans streptococci contains a large group of species of alpha hemolytic Streptococci. The name viridans mean "green color" which was derived from Latin word "viridis" due to their ability to cause green coloration on blood agar plates, "alpha hemolysis" characteristic. They do not grow on media containing more than 6.5% of NaCl. They are optochin resistant hence can be differentiated from alpha hemolytic *S. pneumoniae*. Also, they are negative on bile aesculin agar, therefore they can be differentiated from positive species of *Enterococci*. Their ability of producing bacteriocins and hydrogen peroxide plays significant role by preventing colonization of many pathogens in place where they resides. *S. mutans, S. anginosus, S. mitis, S. oralis, S. sobrinus* and *S. intermedius* are some of the viridans streptococci. They are associated for number of infections including endocarditis, dental carries, abscesses, and occasionally bacteremia [32, 33].

Enterococci

Enterococci are Gram-positive cocci, catalase negative, non-motile, non-spore forming, and facultative anaerobes. They are usually appear in pairs (diplococci) or very short chains. *Enterococci* were once classified as *Streptococci* in the Lancefield group D, until 1984 when they were assigned another genus. There are about 17 different species in the genus *Enterococci* however only two species; *E. faecalis* and *E. faecium* are very common commensals of human gastrointestinal tract. *Enterococci* gives positive results to bile aesculin test which differentiate them from *Viridans streptococci* which are bile aesculin negative. Because of their ability to survive adverse environmental conditions such as extreme temperatures, dry surfaces and sometimes they can live in poorly reconstituted antiseptic agents, makes them be potential pathogens in healthcare associated infections (HCAIs) and causing numbers of outbreaks. They are causing HCAIs mainly among immunocompromised patients. Mostly, septicemia, endocarditis, surgical (wound) site infections, urinary tract infections, enterococcal meningitis, and intra-abdominal infections are implicated by *Enterococci*.

Pathogenesis and virulence factors of *Enterococci*

For *Enterococci* to be able to cause infections, they have to initially attach themselves on tissue surface they are infecting, escape host immunity reactions and then destroy host tissues. This phenomenon is achieved via numbers of virulence factors in Enterococci species explained below;

Surface adhesins; this cell-wall anchored collagen-binding MSCRAMM-AcE (microbial surface binding component recognizing adhesive matrix molecule adhesins of collagen from *Enterococci*) is responsible for adherence to collagen surfaces such as heart valves and aortic tissues of humans. MSCRAMM-AcE, structurally and functionally relates staphylococcal Can adhesins [34, 35].

Enterococcal fibronectin binding protein A (EfbA); another adhesins found on surfaces of Enterococci which facilitate adhesion to human fibronectin of the cardiac endothellum. When cardiac tissues are damaged the risk of Enterococci adhesion increases as fibronectin is exposed [34, 35].

Biofilm formation; this multicellular microcolony is formed when planktonic bacteria stick to one another and to the surface using extracellular polymeric substances including extracellular polysaccharides, lipids, protein and DNA [35, 36].

Hemolysin; it is a cytolitic protein which lyses human red blood cells. By using model animals, Enterococci strains with hemolysin were more virulent with increased severity of infection and mortality of 55% than those Enterococci strains without hemolysin [34, 35].

Gelatinase; this extracellular zinc metalloprotease enzyme is capable of hydrolyzing human hemoglobin, gelatin, casein, collagen and complement components C3 and C3a. Using animal models, gelatinase was found to be associated with endocarditis however it was not significant [34, 35].

Gram-positive bacilli (rods)

Gram-positive bacilli are rod shaped bacteria resist decolonization with Gram stain decolorizer. There are five genera of medical importance Gram-positive bacilli; *Clostridium, Bacillus, Listeria, Gardenella* and *Corynebacterium*. Members of *Bacillus, Listeria* and *Corynebacterium* are aerobes while members of *Clostridium* are anaerobes. Moreover, *Bacillus* and *Clostridium* are spore formers while the rest are non-spore formers.

Listeria

Genus Listeria contains Gram-positive bacilli, non-spore formers, catalase positive, beta hemolytic, and glucose fermenters species. All Listeria species exhibit "tumbling" motility between 20^0C and 25^0C only, they are poorly or non-motile between 35^0C and 37^0C. Recently, Listeria contains the following species; *L. monocytogenes, L. ivanovii, L. innocua, L. grayi, L. welshimeri, L. marthii, L. seeligeri, L. rocourtiae, L. fleischmannii* and *L. weihenstephanensis* [37, 38].

Listeria monocytogenes

L. monocytogenes is facultative intracellular pathogen that is divided into 13 serovars (serotypes) depending on flagella (H) and somatic (S) antigens. Almost all human listeriosis cases are caused by 1/2a, 1/2b and 4b among 1/2a, 1/2b, 1/2c, 3a, 3b, 3c, 4a, 4ab, 4b/4Bx, 4c, 4d, 4e and 7 serovars. Also, *L. monocytogenes* is associated with almost all cases of human listeriosis among others Listeria species [37].

Commonly, people become asymptomatic carriers of *L. monocytogenes* in the gastro-intestines through ingestion of contaminated food. However, some may develop acute gastroenteritis with fever of which symptoms manifest in 1 to 2 days after ingestion. Majority of pregnant women develops acute symptomatic infection with Listeria than non-pregnant women. Through ingestion of amniotic fluid in utero, hematogenous transmission via placenta from maternal circulation and ascending of bacteria from colonized or infected vagina, neonates may become infected. Mostly, intra-uterine infections among neonates are septicemia and meningitis. Early onset of listeriosis among neonates, presents with the following signs and

28

symptoms; cardiopulmonary distress, hepatosplenomegaly, skin rashes and central nervous system signs with mortality rate between 30% and 60% [9, 37].

Pathogenesis and virulence factors of L. monocytogenes

This bacteria is using *internalins* (internalins A and internalins B) to attach itself on human cells whereby with this interaction, phagocytosis of bacteria by host cells is induced mainly by non-phagocytic cells. Internalins A attaches human epithelial cells through E-cadherin receptors while internalins B attaches complement component C1g through globular portion receptor. After phagocytosis, before lysosome fuses with phagosome, bacteria produces *listeriolysin O* (a pore-forming hemolysin similar to streptolysin O of GAS) and other phospholipases that enables bacteria to escape its death. *ActA*, bacterial surface protein is then produced to promote formation of actin "tails" which enables extrusion and fusion with another human cells hence directly spreading between cells [37, 39].

Corynebacterium

Corynebacterium, these Gram-positive bacilli belonging to the class *Actinobacteria*, are pleomorphic, catalase positive, non-motile, non-spore formers, club-shaped with classical description of "picket fence" and "Chinese letters" on Gram stained smears [39, 40]. *Corynebacterium* are non-acid fast bacteria however they contains mycolic acid in their cell walls. Among all Corynebacterium species, *C. diphtheria* a causative agent of deadly disease known as diphtheria, is of medical important to human. Other *Corynebacterium* species include; *Corynebacterium amycolatum* and *Corynebacterium jeikeium* (known human normal flora of the skin), and *Corynebacterium pseudotuberculosis, Corynebacterium ulcerans* and *Corynebacterium xerosis* (considered as zoonotic agents) [40, 41].

Pathogenesis and virulence factors of C. diphtheria

A heat stable diphtheria toxin contains two fragments, A and B. Fragment B binds and toxin enters susceptible cells by receptors-mediated endocytosis and then fragment A catalyses the transfer of adenosine diphosphate ribose (ADPR) from nicotinamide adenine dinucleotide (NAD) to elongation factor 2. This process of adenoribosylation in affected cells, inactivates elongated factor 2 and inhibit protein synthesis. Thereafter, necrotic and neurotoxic effect of the toxin takes place. Sore throat, malaise and difficult in swallowing are the initial symptoms of the infection which is later followed with diphtheritic pseudomembrane which is the accumulation of bacteria and inflammatory cells on the site of infection. If progress to laryngeal, obstruction of larynx and airways takes place thereafter toxaemia results from multiplying organisms resulting to myocarditis and congestive heart failure [37, 42].

Bacillus

The genus *Bacillus* includes all large Gram-positive rod shaped bacteria that are spore-formers that are either aerobes or anaerobes. They are ubiquitous in a wide range of environment, dust, soil, and water. The genus comprises of more than 70 species whereby *B. anthracis* and *B. cereus* are of medical importance.

Bacillus anthracis

This large Gram-positive rods, are catalase positive, exists in chains, spore forming and the only obligate (can grow aerobically or anaerobically) pathogen in the genus *Bacillus*. It can exist as spores (dormant) and vegetative (actively replicating), and it cause a deadly disease known as anthrax. Bacteria form spores (which may live for decades) when exposed to non-conducive environment where no nutrients and then spores germinates when found environment rich in nutrients [43]. From Greek work, "anthrakis" meaning "coal" this bacteria got its name because of its ability to cause coal-like cutaneous eschars [43]. It was a zoonotic pathogen infecting wild and domestic animals; deer, antelope, goats and cattle which was acquired during grazing from contaminated vegetation but recently it is affecting humans who come into contacts with contaminated environment or infected animals. After ingestion of spores it takes 3 to 7 days for clinical symptoms to presents. Depending on the mode of entry, human anthrax is divided into; cutaneous anthrax (through skin breach), oropharyngeal/gastrointestinal anthrax (through mucosa), injectional anthrax (through injections) and inhalational anthrax (through inhalation of spores or aerosols containing bacteria) [37, 43]. Of which, about 95% to 99% of global human anthrax cases are cutaneous anthrax and mainly occurring from Asia, Eastern Europe and Africa [37].

Pathogenesis and virulence factors of *B. anthracis*

30

At entry site, spores germinate into vegetative bacteria and then multiply extracellularly while producing capsules and toxins. If inhaled, they are deposited at the alveolar spaces where they are taken to mediastinal lymph nodes by lymph vessels. Vegetative bacteria are then enters blood stream causing severe septicemia while producing exotoxins and final death occurs [43].

There are major three virulence factors of B. anthracis namely; 83kDa protective antigen (PA), 89kDa edema factor (EF, calmodulin-dependent adenylate cyclase) and 83kDa lethal factor (LF, zinc metalloprotease) which are encoded by virulence plasmids; PXO1 and PXO2 [43]. On target cells, PA binds tumor endothelial marker 8 (TEM 8) and capillary morphogenesis protein 2 (CMG 2) and then it undergoes proteolytic breaking into 22kDa and 63kDa fragments. 63kDa PA fragments polymerizes with alike fragments to form heptamer with a ring shape resulting to pores on cell membranes of target cells. Each 63kDa PA monomer in a heptamer acts as adhesin to bind LF and EF to form LF-PA and EF-PA complexes then enters target cells by endocytosis. Within target cells (phagosome), due to acidic PH, complexes dissociate to release free LF and EF. Then, LF hydrolyzes protein kinase (dealing with transduction of intracellular signals), inhibits synthesis of macromolecules and promotes apoptosis in macrophages. EF inhibits phagocytosis process and deregulates cytokines production by increasing intracellular CAMP levels [37]. Moreover, localized swelling of cutaneous anthrax, is thought to be a result of EF [9].

Bacillus cereus

This soil habitating Gram-positive bacillus is facultative anaerobe, motile, catalase positive, utilizes citrate and grows between 10^0C and 50^0C. They can also be found contaminating agricultural and dairy products. Furthermore, most strains of B. cereus can grow on extreme low temperature therefore refrigeration of food does not prevent food from spoilage. B. cereus is responsible with acute and self-limiting gastroenteritis "food poisoning infection" that is associated with eating contaminated vegetable dishes, cakes, meat, sauces, puddings and salads with emetic toxin or enterotoxigenic B. cereus [44]. There are two types of food poisoning documented, short incubation symptoms with incubation period of 1-6 hours and symptoms of nausea, vomiting and abdominal cramps, and long incubation symptoms with incubation period of 8-16 hours and symptoms of nausea, abdominal crumps, tenesmus and profuse watery diarrhea. *B. cereus* is not limited to gastroenteritis, but it can cause other non-gastrointestinal infections including bacteremia, ocular infections, endocarditis, skin and soft tissue infections and bones infections.

Pathogenesis and virulence factors of *B. cereus* in causing gastroenteritis

The bacteria have heat labile enterotoxins; two protein complexes (hemolysin (HBL) enterotoxin and nonhemolytic (NHE) enterotoxin) and two enterotoxic proteins (enterotoxic T and cytotoxin K). HBL have hemolytic, cytolic and dermanecrotic properties. HBL causes hemolysis of erythrocytes by promoting pores formation on cell membranes resulting to leakage of cytoplasmic contents. Also, HBL increases vascular permeability resulting to accumulation of extracellular fluids. NHE, a cytotoxic and dermonecrotic, also increases cellular membrane permeability.

Clostridium

Clostridia are saprophytic Gram-positive bacilli (sometimes appear as Gram-negative bacilli) are anaerobic spore forming found in environment and decomposing animals and plants. They play important role in decomposition of dead matters, as soon after death they invade tissues and blood circulation. *C. tetani, C. botulinum, C. perfringens* and *C. difficile* are species clostridia of medical importance.

C. difficile

Also known as *C. diff*, is Gram-positive bacilli which is anaerobic, motile, spore-forming, toxin-forming known to cause increasing incidences of healthcare associated infectious diarrhea and fulminant colitis which is associated with long term exposure to broad spectrum antibiotics. *C. diff* infections are abbreviated as CDI. Sometimes, can invade blood stream and cause life-threatening sepsis. Fulminant colitis, caused by hypervirulent strains known as *C. diff* NAP-1/027 or NAB1/B1/027, is very fatal with mortality of 80% and sometimes may require colectomy. Fulminant colitis presents with diarrhea, fever, abdominal distension, diffuse abdominal pain, leukocytosis (~40,000 leukocytes/µl), hypoalbuminemia, severe lactic acidosis [45].

Pathogenesis and virulence factors of *C. diff*

CDI-mediated by two enterotoxins; toxin A (TcdA) which is enterotoxin and toxin B (TcdB) which is cytotoxin. It has been documented that, strains of *C. diff* lacking both TcdA and TcdB are non-pathogenic. Toxins enter cells of the gastrointestinal tract (GIT) through receptors by modification of Rho-proteins (glutamyl transpeptidase-binding proteins). Entry of toxins into GIT cells result to increased permeability of intestines therefore secretion of fluids (mediated by toxin A) and increased intense inflammations of the colon (mediated by toxin B). As a result, intracellular tight junction is lost hence secretory diarrhea, inflammations and cell death [46, 47].

C. tetani

This obligatory anaerobe is motile, slender, have large terminal spore making it looks like "drum stick". On sheep blood agar it gives thin spreading film growth characteristic. Spores of *C. tetani* are resistant to boiling (100^0C) for 3 hours, dry heating (160^0C) for 1 hour, 5% phenol for 2 weeks but 1% iodine in water is effective within hours however glutaraldehyde disinfectants are said to be sporicidal. These bacteria cause dramatic "tetanus" disease which is characterized by spastic contractions of voluntary muscles and hyperreflexia. Incubation period for tetanus is 3-21 days. Tetanus is a result of bacterial spores contaminating wound from puncture, injury or laceration however few cases of neonatal tetanus have been associated with contaminated umbilical cord. Penetrating injuries/wounds and mixed aerobic bacterial infections deprive oxygen to low oxygen tension which favors germinating condition for spores to vegetative cells of *C. tetani* which multiplies and produce toxins.

Pathogenesis and virulence factors of *C. tetani*

C. tetani produces two toxins; tetanolysin (oxygen-labile hemolysin) and tetanospasmin (neurotoxin). Bacteria stay at the site of infection but toxins will be absorbed and circulating blood facilitates transmission of toxins to all nerves of the body. The autolysis of bacteria releases tetanospasmin which travels to central nervous system (CNS) from nerve endings of peripheral lower motor neurons that activate voluntary muscles. In the CNS, toxin blocks inhibitory impulses to motor neurons by binding to gangliosides. When attaches binding sites at myoneural junctions, tetanospasmin inhibit acetylcholine release as occur with botulinum toxin. Nerve endings of inhibitory GABAergic and/or gylcinergic neurons dealing with lower motor neurons activities take up toxin through synapses. In inhibitory terminals, toxin cleaves VAMP (vesicle associated membrane protein) so inhibiting the release of GABA and glycine. All these result to denervation of lower motor neurons leading to their hyperactivity which increase muscle rigidity and spasms. Then, patients experiences painful muscles contraction with backward arching due to contraction of back muscles and lockjaw "trismus" due to difficult in opening jaws. Also, patient may experience rigidity and spasms of laryngeal and respiratory muscles resulting to respiratory failure [48].

Tetanus should be taken as emergency medicine which requires immediate hospitalization and treatment with 3000-6000 units of human tetanus immunoglobulin (HTI). Also, aggressive management of wound by cleaning and left it open and loose with administration of antibiotics; metronidazole or penicillin [48, 49].

C. botulinum

C. botulinum is Gram-positive bacilli (rod shaped), spore-forming, obligate anaerobe which is divided into I, II, III and IV groups according to physiological differences. These bacteria are the causative agent of botulism a neuroparalytic syndrome. Depending on mode of entry/infection and age, there is foodborne botulism, infant botulism, wound botulism, inhalational botulism and rarely waterborne botulism and botulism of unknown origin. *Foodborne botulism* happen by ingestion of pre-formed toxins in contaminated food especially vegetables and fruits. Early symptoms of this type include fatigue, weakness, blurred vision, dry mouth, difficult in speaking and swallowing. Sometimes diarrhea, vomiting, abdominal swelling and constipation occur. Lastly, flaccid paralysis which may results to respiratory failure happen. *Infant botulism* affects infants aged below 6 months whereby they ingest bacterial spore that germinate to produce toxins in the gut. Mothers are restricted from feeding their infants honey till the age of 1 year as some rare cases of spores-contaminating honey have been reported. Infant botulism presents with constipation, loss of appetite, striking loss of head control, weakness and altered cry. *Wound botulism* happen when spores get into wound where they find favorable anaerobic condition for germinating to vegetative bacteria which release toxins. But cases of wound botulism are very rare. *Inhalational botulism*, very rare, occurs accidentally or intentionally when individuals inhale aerosols-containing toxins during bioterrorism [50].

Pathogenesis and virulence factors of *C. botulinum*

C. botulinum produces deadliest botulinum neurotoxin (BoNT) which comprises with two chains (100kDa heavy chain and 50kDa light chain) linked by disulfide bridge. Recently, eight serotypes, A, B, C, D, E, F, G and H are identified of which BoNT/A and BoNT/B are more potent serotypes. Mostly, single strain of *C. botulinum* produces only one serotype but dual serotypes-producing strains have been reported. In bloodstream, BoNT goes to voluntary motor and autonomic neuromuscular junctions (NMJs) where they bind to presynaptic nerve terminals. Following endocytosis facilitated by heavy chain is cleavage of the light chain in cytosol. Thereafter, serotype-specific targets of the SNARE (SNAP-25, VAMP or syntaxin) polypeptide complexes are cleaved after being targeted by light chain. After cleavage of these complexes, presynaptic acetylcholine (Ach) release is blocked and muscles contraction is inhibited resulting to flaccid paralysis [51].

C. perfringens

C. perfringens is a large Gram-positive bacilli which is ubiquitous to the environment (soil, food, feces and sewage systems), non-motile, heat resistant spore-former, normal flora to humans and animals gut, and grow well at 42°C as its doubling time is reduced to 8 minutes. This bacteria is significant causative agent of a foodborne disease "food poisoning", gas gangrene and rarely cases of highly mortality (>60%) septicemia, antibiotic associated diarrhea (5%-15% cases) and fatal enteritis necroticans [52-54].

Strains of *C. perfringens* are classified into five different toxinotypes; A, B, C, D and E depending on their ability of toxins production of four different types namely, alpha (CPA), beta (CPB), epsilon (ETX) and iota (ITX). However strains of *C. perfringens* are not limited to production of only one type of toxin, some produces even three different types for example *C. perfringens* toxinotype B is able to produce CPA, CPB and ETX toxins [52].

Pathogenesis and virulence factors of *C. perfringens* in causing gas gangrene

It is known that, *C. perfringens* cannot escape host immune response such as phagocytosis, therefore to achieve gas gangrene (clostridial myonecrosis) formation there should be some risk factors. These factors include presence of dead tissues, pyogenic infection, and a clot of blood, oozing fluid and foreign bodies such as soil on wound. Other risk factors are diabetes and old age. All together these factors are causing poor supply of oxygen to the wound and a reduction of E_h resulting to impaired intraleucocytic bactericidal and phagocytic mechanisms. Therefore, providing very conducing environment for *C. perfringens'* spores to germinate into vegetative bacilli and start producing toxins and gas, with further impairment in local blood supply. Extreme toxaemia resulting to shock, severe hypotension, multiple organ failure, coma and finally death [9, 55, 56].

Pathogenesis and virulence factors of *C. perfringens* in causing enteritis necroticans

Enteritis necroticans also known as "pigbel" caused by toxins of *C. perfringens* toxinotype C is a segmental gangrene of the bowel which is characterized with inflammation, ischemic necrosis of jejunum, and hemorrhagic. Under specific dietary conditions mainly involving eating of pre-cooked food, mostly meat that allows survival of bacteria along with proteinase inhibitor containing food such as sweet potato. *C. perfringens* beta (CPB) toxin produced in small intestines induces necrotizing enteritis [57, 58].

Pathogenesis and virulence factors of *C. perfringens* in causing food poisoning

C. perfringens toxinotype A is the common food poisoning agent worldwide however very few strains (less than 5%) are capable of producing enterotoxin responsible for food poisoning. Sporulation of *C. perfringens* toxinotype A in small intestine produces enterotoxin while vegetative bacteria are forming spores. Released enterotoxin induces acute diarrhea and abdominal cramps which is self-limiting within 12-24 hours however in other cases it can go to 3 days. Condition may become very severe and prolonged among elderly and immunocompromised individuals. Severity of infection include necrosis of the intestines, peritonitis and septicemia however mortality is very low. Long waiting of serving of large quantity of food prepared hours before at restaurants and catering is the most factor associated with food poisoning with *C. perfringens* toxinotype A [59].

Gardenella

Gardenella, anaerobic coccobacilli, non-spore forming, vaginal normal flora, and having Gram-positive like type of cell wall because its peptidoglycan layer in its cell wall is very thin compared to other Gram-positive bacteria is the significant causative agent of discharging bacterial vaginosis (BV). Formerly, this bacterium was known as *Hemophillus vaginalis* or *Corybacterium vaginale*, but later in 1980 it was described as *Gardenella vaginalis*. These bacteria, together with *Mobiluncus* spp are isolated from about 97% of women diagnosed with discharging BV however *Gardenella vaginalis* may be isolated from males' sexual partners. The pathogenesis of *Mobiluncus* spp in causing BV is not clearly understood. BV infection increases the risk of acquiring other sexually transmitted infections (STIs), because BV is also sexually transmitted. Also, *Gardenella vaginalis* has been assocociated with preterm birth among infected pregnant women. *Lactobacillus* species predominate vagina niche, when *Gardenella vaginalis* starts to overgrow and predominate *Lactobacillus* species, is when BV happens [60, 61].

Pathogenesis and virulence of *G. vaginalis* in causing bacterial vaginosis (BV)

First *G. vaginalis* compete successful with *Lactobacillus* species for attachment to epithelial cells of the vagina using adhesin factors. Then producing vaginolysin (pore-forming toxin), a cholesterol-dependent cytolysin that affects only human cells. This toxin initiates complex signaling cascades causing lysis of target cells hence bacteria's virulence [60].

Gram negative bacteria

Enterobacteriaceae

Family Enterobacteriaceae are Gram-negative rods, non-spore forming, catalase positive, cytochrome oxidase negative, glucose fermenters, able to reduce nitrate to nitrite, facultative anaerobes and most are motile. Because of their natural habitat which is humans and animals gastrointestinal tract, they have given names like enteric bacteria and enterobacteria. This genus is comprising with species know to be true pathogens (*Salmonella* species, *Shigella* species and *Yersinia* species) and opportunistic pathogens causing human diseases such as sepsis, diarrhea, meningitis, urinary tract infections, pneumonia, osteomyelitis and many others. Genera of medical importance include; Escherichia, Klebsiella, Enterobacter, Citrobacter, Salmonella, Shigella, Proteus, Vibrio, Serratia, Morganella, Yersinia, and Providencia species.

Lactose fermenting Gram-negative bacteria
Genus Escherichia

Escherichia coli (*E. coli*) are the significant causative agents of different human diseases among all other species in the genus Escherichia. *E. coli* is the predominant aerobic normal flora of human and animals' guts. Strains of *E. coli* are Gram-negative rods, motile, cytochrome oxidase negative, non-spore forming, catalase positive, reduces nitrate to nitrite, ferment lactose sugar and produces indole from tryptophan. However some strain (very few) of *E. coli*, does not produce indole (~2%), utilizes citrate (~1%), produce urease enzyme (~1%), non-motile (~5%), and does not ferment lactose (~5%). From DNA-DNA recombination studies, *Escherichia* and *Shigella* species belongs to the same tribe therefore this explains variable characteristics of *E. coli* strains.

Antigenic structure and virulence factors of *E. coli*

Antigenically, *E. coli* contains lipopolysaccharide (LPS) O, flagella (H) and capsule (K), of which O and H antigens are routinely used for serotyping these bacteria. K antigens, specifically K1 are reported to be associated with virulence particularly in causing meningitis among neonates. Also, in absence of specific antibodies to K antigens alone or K and O antigens, K antigens inhibit bactericidal activity of complement and phagocytes against bacteria. *E. coli* strains produce vast number of toxins which are used as virulence factors. Toxins include enterotoxin, shiga type toxin, shiga like toxin, and hemolysin. These toxins are discussed below under specific description of pathogenesis of pathogenic *E. coli*.

Enterotoxigenic *E. coli* (ETEC)

Enterotoxigenic *E. coli* (ETEC) is the causative agent of traveler's diarrhea and weanling diarrhea and known producer of secretory enterotoxins. Recently, 18 serotypes are common; O6, O8, O15, O20, O25, O27, O63, O78, O80, O85, O92, O115, O128ac, O139, O148, O153, O159 and O167. Enterotoxins, two types existing; heat labile (LT) and heat stable (ST) toxins are produced by ETEC strains responsible for causing watery diarrhea. Two forms of LT and ST exists, LT-I and LT-II, and ST-I and ST-II respectively. ST-I is a plasmid encoded, however the same plasmid may be encoding other genes responsible for LTs and antibiotics resistance. ETEC produce either one type or both. Both types contain one alpha subunit for toxic enzymatic activity and five beta subunit for binding target cells in the bowel. ETEC strains binds to epithelial cells of the small intestine using fimbriae via colonization factor antigens (CFAs) or coli surface antigens (CSAs). Binding of LTs on specific receptors on epithelial cells of the bowel, they stimulate the release of adenylate cyclase enzyme causing an increased production of cyclic adenosine monophosphate (cAMP). STs stimulates production of cGMP, however it is not clearly understood. On the other hand, cGMP also stimulates production of cAMP. This resulting to ion imbalance because of altered activities of sodium and chloride transporters leading to fluid accumulation in the bowel therefore watery diarrhea usually without mucus, pus or blood [62, 63].

Enteropathogenic *E. coli* (EPEC)

EPEC a causative agent of a condition known as "attaching and effacing" lesions (A/E lesions), usually among infants (infantile enteritis) characterized by malaise, vomiting, low grade fever and watery diarrhea with eminent amount of mucus but without blood. EPEC common serogroups are O26, O55, O86, O111, O114, O119, O125, O126, O127, O128, O142 and O158. EPEC strains, specifically serogroup O26 have been associated with production of verocytotoxin. However, in general, no toxins associated with EPEC have been detected [62].

Eneteroinvasive *E. coli* (EIEC)

EIEC, this causative agent of dysentery shares the same pathogenesis as *Shigella dysentriae*. Common serogroups of EIEC include, O28ac, O29, O78, O112ac, O115, O124, O136, O148, O153, O159 and O167. Pathogenicity of EIEC depends on chromosomal genes encoding for aerobactin-mediated iron-sequestering system and long chains LPS [9, 37]. EIEC dysentery is characterized with mucus, blood and a lot of leukocytes [37].

Enterohemorrhagic *E. coli* (EHEC)

EHEC also known as Verocytotoxin-producing *E. coli* (VTEC) was discovered in 1977 with ability of producing protein cytotoxic toxin (Verocytotoxin) for vero cells of the kidney. This discovery linked EHEC with hemorrhagic colitis and haemolytic uraemic syndrome (HUS). Moreover, EHEC is also an etiological cause of A/E lesions like EPEC. Common serogroups of EHEC include O26,

O111, O112ac, O124, O136, O143, O144, O152, O157 and O164, however O157 is far more common than others.

E. coli O157:H7 is the major global health concern associated with waterborne and foodborne "life-threatening" disease of hemorrhagic colitis, HUS and thrombotic thrombocytopenic purpura (TTP). HUS may progress to acute renal failure, a systemic morbidity. Interestingly, farm ruminant animals are natural carriers of E. coli O157:H7. Verocytotoxin (VT) produced by E. coli O157:H7 is Shiga like toxin produced by Shigella dysentriae type 1. The difference between VT from E. coli O157:H7 and S. dysentriae type 1 is the location of encoding genes, in E. coli O157:H7 these genes are carried by lambda-like bacteriophage while in S. dysentriae type 1 the genes are carried on chromosome. VT causing hemorrhagic diarrhea/colitis by binding on and sloughing off of intestinal mucosa cells. Furthermore, VT causes vasculitis due to its systemic effects on vascular endothelial cells. Later on, HUS, abdominal pain and sometimes with TTP become obvious. Initiation of inflammatory cascades by VT results to aggregation of leukocytes and platelets, hemolysis, formation of microthrombi and apoptosis of affected cells. Vulnerability of renal glomeruli to microthrombi results to renal failure/dysfunction [64, 65].

Enteroaggregative E. coli (EAEC/EAggEC)

EAEC got its name due to its ability of adhering on epithelial cells in an "aggregative" or "stacked brick" pattern. EAEC, marked for its etiological cause of chronic, mucoid, watery, secretory diarrhea especially among malnourished children. Pathogenesis of EAEC in causing diarrhea is not clearly understood, but its ability to adhere to HEp-2 is presumed to have something with pathogenesis. However, some strains produce LT-toxin, ST-like toxin, hemolysin and aggregative adherence fimbriae (AAFs) [66-68].

Uropathogenic E. coli (UPEC)

UPEC pathotypes are considered as the main causative agents of urinary tract infections (UTIs) of over 80% especially those acquired in the community (CA-UTIs). Recently, four phylogroups of UPEC have been identified, A, B1, B2 and D based on expression of virulence factors and genomic Pathogenicity Island (PAI). The pathogenesis of UPEC in causing UTI include colonization of periurethral, vaginal and urethral cells; ascending to bladder; adherence to epithelial cells of the bladder; form biofilm; invasion and replication in the bladder; and ascending to and colonization of kidney. Colonization of kidneys by UPEC increases the risk of development to urosepsis if effective treatment will delay [69, 70].

UPEC attach and colonizes urinary tract mucosa by using pili, fimbriae (type 1 fimbriae, P fimbriae and aggregative fimbriae) and adhesins (Dr/Afa, TosA and FdeC). Pili and fimbriae are not limited to adhesion only, but help bacteria to survive and evade host immune response. Furthermore, UPEC uses different toxins to play its significant role of effective virulent strain in causing UTIs by destroying host cells, evade immune responses and for self-propagation. HlyA (α-hemolysin), pore-forming toxin lyses host erythrocytes and other nucleated cells when present in high concentration however in its low concentration still it can promote exfoliation of epithelial cells and induces apoptosis of target cells. Using cytotoxic necrotizing factor 1 (CNF 1), UPEC escapes phagocytosis by polymorph nuclear cells and promotes apoptosis of epithelial cells of the bladder. Another toxin is "secreted autotransporter toxin" SAT, having cytopathic activity, it damages host tissues hence increasing propagation of UPEC. Also, SAT facilitates entry of UPEC into bloodstream resulting to urosepsis. UPEC have ability of destroying DNA of target cells resulting to their death through its production of cytolethal distending toxin (CDT). Other virulence factors by UPEC are siderophores, aerobactin, enterobactin, LPS and salmochelin [69, 71-76].

Genus *Klebsiella*

These capsulated Gram-negative rods are non-motile, lactose fermenters, catalase producers, negative to cytochrome oxidase, and facultative anaerobes. *Klebsiella* species shares the same tribe (*Klebsielleae*) with *Enterobacter*, *Hafnia* and *Serratia*. Klebsiella species produces significant capsular (polysaccharides in nature, resembling K antigens of *E. coli*) materials when grown on culture media containing carbohydrates. Colonies of *Klebsiella* species on culture media are greyish-white, luxuriant and mucoid. Recently six species have been identified, *K. pneumoniae*, *K. oxytoca*, *K. granulomatis*, *K. singaporensis*, *K. ulba* and *K. variicola*.

In 2001, bacteriologists based on sequences of 16S rRNA and *rpo*B genes evidence, proposed a division of genus Klebsiella into two genus named *Raoultella* and *Klebsiella* and *K. oxytoca* is a monophyletic taxon. From their findings, they concluded that, *Klebsiella* is heterogeneous comprising of three phyletic clusters, I, II and III. *K. granulomatis* and *K. pneumoniae* subspecies *pneumoniae, rhinoscleromatis*, and *ozane* belongs to cluster I. *K. ornithinolytica, K. planticola, K. terrigena* and *K. trevisanii* belongs to cluster II. Cluster III contains only *K. oxytoca* [77]. Herein, two principal species, *K. pneumoniae* and *K. oxytoca* are explained in details.

K. pneumoniae

First this species was named as Friedlander's bacillus after Carl Friedlander in 1882 who isolated it from lungs of patients who died from pneumonia. This encapsulated, gram negative, non-motile bacteria, a typical colonizer of humans' and animals' guts, has been associated with severe hospital acquired pneumonia characterized with multiple abscesses in the lungs. Frequently, patients produce thick, mucoid and brick red sputum described as "currant jelly" as a result of extensive hemorrhage and necrosis of tissues of the lungs. Differently, community acquired pneumonia due to *S. pneumoniae* described "rust" or "blood tinged". Mostly infecting alcoholic, patients with diabetes and those with chronic obstructive pulmonary disease. Although, *K. pneumoniae* can cause other extra-pulmonary infections including urinary tract infections (UTIs), endocarditis, skin and soft tissue infections, septicemia and meningitis in infants [37, 78].

Pathogenesis and virulence factors of *K. pneumoniae*

Initiation of infection by *K. pneumoniae* starts with attachment to host cells using fimbriae such as KPF-28 and adhesins such as CF29K and CS31A. Then, polysaccharide capsule of *K. pneumoniae* plays important roles of protecting these bacteria against actions of complement cascades and opsonization by host immune system. Also, capsule decreases permeability of antibiotics into bacterial cells rendering these strains resistant to multiple antibiotics [79-81]. Production of siderophores helps these bacteria in competition of iron uptake against host cells for its metabolism. The more competent bacteria is in iron uptake, the more virulent and invasive. Urease production benefits uropathogenic *K. pneumoniae* in precipitating inorganic salts resulting to formation of infectious stones in the kidneys by increasing localized pH.

Formation of biofilm makes *K. pneumoniae* less susceptible to killing by antibiotics as it provides resistance in penetrating bacteria cells. Also, biofilm reduces susceptibility of host immune mechanisms against the bacteria [82].

Hypervirulent *K. pneumoniae* (HvKP)

Hypervirulent *K. pneumoniae* abbreviated by HvKP was first reported from Asian Pacific Rim [83]. HvKP have increased ability of iron uptake and production of polysaccharide capsule giving its hypermucoviscous phenotype. HvKP strains can be identified in the laboratory by a simple string test whereby it is positive when touched by inoculating loop away from the plate and gives a string of >5mm in length. Molecular characterization revealed that, HvKP strains harbor *K1*, *K2*, *rmp*A, *rmp*A2, *mag*A and aerobactin virulence-associated genes [84, 85]. Primarily, HvKP is associated with metastatic pyogenic liver abscesses (PLA), metastasizing towards central nervous system, lungs and eyes. Yet, HvKP causes other infections like septicemia. Infections with HvKP are always of poor prognosis and of high mortality rate [85, 86].

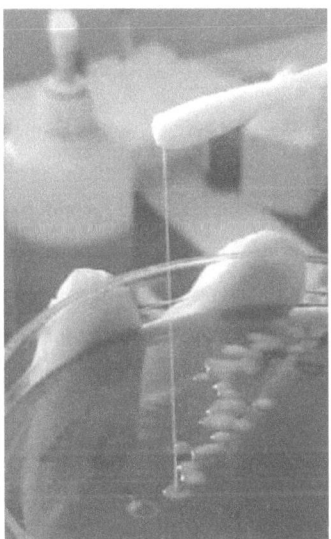

Figure 5: Hypervirulent *K. pneumoniae* (HvKP) showing hypermucoviscous and string test positive, isolated from urine culture on MacConkey agar plate.

K. pneumoniae carbapenemase (KPC)

KPC are K. pneumoniae strains capable of producing plasmid-encoded carbapenemase (eg. KPC, VIM, OXA and NDM) enzymes conferring them resistance to carbapenems (meropenem, imipenem, ertapenem and doripenem) and other beta-lactam antibiotics. KPC is an emerging global health concern with significant increasing mortality rate. About 70% of KPC strains in the CDC database between 1996 and 2008 are multilocus sequence type 258 (ST258) [87-89].

K. oxytoca

First described in 1886 when it was isolated from sour milk hence the origin of its name, "oxytoca". In Greek language, "oxus" means sour and "tokos" means producing. K. oxytoca is closely related to K. pneumoniae but are distinguished by the characteristic of indole production from tryptophan by K. oxytoca. This bacterium has been identified as the causative agent of septicemia, respiratory infections and urinary tract infections among many more. Also, K. oxytoca have acquired different mechanisms of antibiotics resistance including extended spectrum beta lactamase and carbapenemases [90]. In addition, some strains of K. oxytoca produce cytotoxins facilitating their virulence [91, 92].

Genus Enterobacter

In general, Enterobacter species are Gram-negative rods, indole negative, utilizes citrate, motile and reduces nitrate to nitrite. However some strains of E. cloacae are non-motile (~3%), urea positive (~2%) and does not utilize citrate (~2%). Also, some strains of E. aerogenes are non-motile (~5%), does not reduce nitrate to nitrite (~1%) and produces urease enzyme (~50%). Enterobacter species are slightly mucoid on culture media. These variations might be attributed from the fact that, Enterobacter species shares the same tribe with Klebsiella species. Naturally, Enterobacter species can be found colonizing human guts, soil and water. E. cloacae, E. aerogenes and E. sakazakii among other species are of medical importance to humans associated with septicemia, respiratory infections, urinary tract infections (UTIs) and skin and soft tissues infections [93].

Virulence factors of Enterobacter species

Enterobacter species possess vast number of virulence factors facilitating their pathogenesis in causing different infections. These virulence factors include outer membrane protein OmpX, endotoxin LPS, type 1 and 3 fimbriae, enterotoxin similar to ST-I and LT-I from *E. coli*, aerobactin-mediated iron uptake system and sometimes hemolysin [94]. *Enterobacter* species are known to have chromosomal mediated (inducible) ampC beta lactamase genes which confers resistance towards broad-spectrum antibiotics of the beta-lactam types [95].

Enterobacter bugandensis

E. bugandensis (EB-247), described recently (2016) is reported to be associate with neonatal sepsis outbreaks in immediate care units and increased mortality rate in this population [96]. EB-247 equips itself with boundless numbers of virulence factors which contributes to its effective pathogenesis. From different studies, EB-247 found with abilities to produce adhesins, polysaccharide capsule, toxin (colicin E2) and O-antigens (cytokines inducers; interleukin 1 and 6, tumor necrotic factor α and interferon γ). EB-247 strains can form biofilm and contains drug efflux system. Yet, EB-247 strains harbor IncH12 plasmid encoding genes for multiple antibiotics resistance [96-98].

Non-lactose fermenters
Genus *Serratia*

Members of this genus are Gram-negative rods, non-lactose fermenters, motile, non-spore formers, facultative anaerobes and they are ubiquitous in nature (water, soil, plants, showers and toilets) but they are not common colonizers of human guts. Few members of this genus produce "prodigiosin", a red pigment which is obvious on culture media like nutrient agar and Muller Hinton agar. Uniquely, *Serratia* species produces DNase, gelatinase and lipase enzymes which are not common among other members of the family *Enterobacteriaceae*. Commonly, *S. marcescens* and sometimes *S. liquefaciens*, *S. odorifera* and *S. plymuthica* are usually causing opportunistic nosocomial infections, mainly, bloodstream infections (BSIs), urinary tract infections (UTIs), surgical site infections (SSIs), lower respiratory tract infections (LRTIs), endocarditis, meningitis and arthritis [99, 100].

Pathogenesis and virulence factors of *Serratia* species

The pathogenesis mechanism of *Serratia* species in causing human infections is not well understood however some virulence factors have been identified to date. Key virulence factors reported among *Serratia* species include biofilm formation, adhesins (fimbriae), long chain LPS, production of protease enzyme for tissue damaging, hemolysins for iron regulation and production of *E. coli* like verocytotoxin and LT toxins [101, 102]. Additionally, *Serratia* species produces chromosomal mediated ampC beta lactamase enzymes making them naturally resistant to beta-lactam antibiotics [103].

Genus *Citrobacter*

The genus *Citrobacter* are gram-negative rods, reduces nitrate to nitrite, produces indole from tryptophan, utilizes citrate, produces urease enzyme, motile, and non-spore formers. *C. freundii* and *C. koseri* are species of medical importance to humans. Some strains of *C. freundii* do not produce indole (~70%), does not utilize citrate (~20%), does not produce urease enzyme (~50%) and are non-motile (~10%). Generally, members of this genus are none or late lactose fermenters. Citrobacter species are ubiquitous in environment including soil, wastewater, and water and can found in guts of humans and animals. Commonly, members of *Citrobacter* are known to cause osteomyelitis, urinary tract infections (UTIs), arthritis, pulmonary infections, endocarditis and neonatal sepsis and meningitis [104-107].

Pathogenesis and virulence factors of *Citrobacter* species

The pathogenic mechanisms of *Citrobacter* species in causing infections are not well understood. Virulence factors like adhesins (fimbriae) for adherence to host cellular surfaces, biofilm formation which helps in evading host immune defence mechanisms and reduces susceptibility for antibiotics, protease enzyme for damaging of host tissues and production of *E. coli* like verocytotoxin type 2 toxin have been reported among *Citrobacter* species [108]. Furthermore, *Citrobacter* species, mostly, *C. freundii* expresses high levels of inducible ampC beta lactamase enzymes leading to clinical failure with beta-lactam antibiotics therapy [109].

Genus *Proteus*

Proteus species are Gram-negative rods, sulphur producers, urease enzyme producers, motile, non-lactose producers and reduces nitrate to nitrite. Majority of *P. mirabilis* utilizes citrate (~65%) while majority of *P. vulgaris* produces indole from tryptophan (~98%) [37]. Generally, *Proteus* species are normal flora of humans and animals gastrointestinal tract, but can also be found from sewage. They further known as saprophytes as they are commonly found on decaying matters. *Proteus* species are marked by their "swarming" growth characteristic on 5% sheep blood agar, forming concentric rings resulting from their cellular elongation and synthesis of flagellin [110]. *P. mirabilis* and *P. vulgaris* are medically important species of humans' mainly causing opportunistic urinary tract infections (UTIs) among patients with indwelling urinary catheters, diabetic, prostatectomy and benign prostatic hypertrophy [111]. Yet, *Proteus* species can cause chronic supurative otitis media, burn wound infections, endocarditis, meningitis, empyema, osteomyelitis, endophthalmitis and meningoencephalitis [112].

Virulence factors of *Proteus* species for pathogenesis

Proteus species have different virulence factors to facilitate their pathogenesis in causing of infections. They have pili and fimbriae for adhesion to host cells, produces cytotoxic hemolysin which lyses red blood cells and release iron for their metabolisms, produces urease enzymes creating alkalinity environment in the kidneys which promotes formation of struvite stones and produces protease (IgAase) enzymes to evade host immune mechanisms [112, 113]. Also, formation of biofilm helps these bacteria in adhesion on indwelling devices facilitating their colonization and then causing infections [113].

Genus *Salmonella*

These intracellular Gram-negative rods are oxidase negative, catalase positive, non-spore formers, motile using petrichious flagella, facultative anaerobes and produces sulfur [114]. This bacteria can grow at very low temperature as 2-4^{0}C [115]. Named after veterinary surgeon DE Salmon who isolated it from porcine intestine in 1884 and named it as *"Bacillus choleraesuis"* [116]. But later on, in 1900 it was renamed to *"Salmonella choleraesuis"* [114, 117]. To date, there are only two species of *Salmonella*, namely *S. enterica* and *S. bongori*. However *S. enterica* is further divided into six subspecies, *S. enterica* subspecies *enterica*, *S. enterica* subspecies *arizonae*, *S. enterica* subspecies *indica*, *S. enterica* subspecies *diarizonae*, *S. enterica* subspecies *salamae* and *S. enterica* subspecies *houtenae*. *S. enterica* subspecies are further divided into more than 2500 serotypes/serovars based on somatic O antigens, flagella H antigens and Vi capsular antigens [118]. But, it was proposed that, *S. enterica* subspecies should be subgenera resulting to over 2500 *Salmonella* species [114, 119].

Pathogenesis and virulence factors of *Salmonella*

S. enterica subspecies *enterica* serotype *typhi* (*S. typhi*) and *S. enterica* subspecies *enterica* serotype *paratyphi* A and C (*S. paratyphi* A and C) are true pathogens of humans. They are very rarely isolated from animals. These serotypes together with *S. enterica* subspecies *enterica* serotype *typhimurium* are causing gastroenteritis, septicemia, enteric fever, carrier state and focal infections [37]. Gastroenteritis is characterized with diarrhea (mild to fulminant), nausea, and vomiting and low grade fever. Septicemia, this infection lack evidence of gastrointestinal is manifested with a very high grade fever. Enteric fever is linked with gastroenteritis, at first phase it is characterized with constipation and fever of which blood culture become positive while stool culture will be negative and its second phase is characterized diarrhea, blood cultures are negative while stool cultures are positives [37]. Carrier state, about 1% to 5% of individuals previously infected and completely treated become chronic carriers and excretes these bacteria (commonly *S. typhi*) in their feces for more than 1 year. In 1906, Mary Mallon was diagnosed as "healthy carrier" who transmitted this pathogen to several homes she worked as a cook [120, 121]. Focal infections are very rare, but meningitis, osteomyelitis, endocarditis and brain abscesses were reported and mostly been implicated by non-typhi Salmonella [122, 123].

For *Salmonella* to invade and achieve intracellular niche, the following virulence factors play important role. Type 1 secretion system (BapA, SiiE), fimbriae and flagella/flagellin promote adhesion, invasiveness and biofilm formation. T3SS1, this facilitates invasion and survival into host cells, and modulate immune response by AvrA effector which inhibit inflammatory response and prevent apoptosis, and tyrosine phosphate SptP switch off ruffle formation. T3SS2, facilitates survival in macrophages. Superoxide dismutase (SodCl), this protects bacteria from killing by extracellular reactive oxygen species. Also, *Salmonella* serotypes produces siderophores (enterobactin and salmochelin) for iron uptake system [124].

Genus *Shigella*

Shigella, causative agent of blood stained mucopurulent diarrhea "dysentery" are Gram-negative rods, non-motile, non-spore formers, does not produce sulphur and reduces nitrate to nitrite. *Shigella* species are known as non-lactose fermenters but about 1%, 1% and 2% of serogroup B, serogroup C and serogroup D ferment lactose respectively [37]. Also, *Shigella* species are very sensitive to direct sunlight and oxygen of which long exposure kills them therefore stool specimens should be cultured within two hours after collection or put in transport media such as Cary Blair [125]. In this case, *Shigella* species are known as fastidious organisms [125]. The name *Shigella* was named after Kiyoshi Shiga a Japanese bacteriologist who discovered this bacteria in 1897 [126].

Shigella are divided into major four serogroups; A (*S. dysentriae*, contains 15 serotypes), B (*S. flexneri*, contains 8 serotypes), C (*S. boydii*, contains 19 serotypes) and D (*S. sonnei*, contain only 1 serotype) [127, 128]. Serogroups A, B and C are physiologically and biochemically similar hence combined to "*Shigella* serogroups A, B and C" by CDC. Dysentery caused by *Shigella* serogroups A, B and C is more severe than that caused by *S. sonnei* (serogroup D). Also, *S. dysentriae* 1 has been associated with hemolytic uraemic syndrome which always results into hemolytic anaemia, thrombocytopenia and acute renal failure.

Bacillary dysentery

This enteric infectious disease is characterized by fever, abdominal pain, tenesmus and diarrhea containing blood and/or mucus. Bacillary dysentery is still a global public health concern with about 165 million annual cases and 1.1 million deaths globally. This disease is very infectious with as low as 10-100 bacterial infectious dose enough to initiate infection to healthy person. It is transmitted via fecal-oral route through contaminated food, water and hands or personal-to-personal contact. The disease is prevalent in countries with low income and facilitated by poor hygiene and overcrowded populations [129-131].

Pathogenesis and virulence factors of *Shigella*

Shigella invades intestinal epithelium by ruffling M-cells and induces its own endocytosis while escaping endocytic vacuole. Then, they are spreading from cell to cell by using cell cytoskeleton actin in which they also invade macrophages and epithelial cells. Their invasion in macrophages induces apoptosis while in epithelial cells they first multiply before inducing death of the infected epithelial cells. Death of macrophages and epithelial cells induces intense immune response mostly release of polymorph nuclear cells (can be seen in stool specimens under microscope) resulting to bleeding and formation of abscesses. To achieve all these, Shigella equipped with virulence factors. Some of those virulence factors include LPS which triggers host immune and inflammatory responses that facilitates bacterial adhesion and invasion; IpaB which binds CD44 promotes bacteria invasion into epithelial cells; IpaC this induces cytoskeletal rearrangement for micropinocytic uptake of bacteria; Shigella enterotoxins 1 and 2 promotes fluid secretion in duodenum and Shiga toxin is known to have neurotoxic properties [132].

Genus *Vibrio*

Bacteria species in this genus are curved (comma shaped) Gram-negative rods, facultative anaerobes, non-spore forming, oxidase positive and motile by using polar flagella. These species are ubiquitous to marine and aquatic environment hence colonizing crabs, prawns and fishes. Unusual to other genus in the family *Enterobacteriaceae*, *Vibrio* have two distinct chromosomes of different origin [133]. *V. cholerae*, *V. parahemolyticus*, *V. alginolyticus* and *V. vulnificus* are human pathogenic species. Apart from *V. cholera* (causative agent of cholera), others are termed as non-cholera species. Non-cholera species causes vibriosis, a mild and self-limiting gastroenteritis which can be transmitted via contaminated water, eating of undercooked seafood and person-to-person contacts [134]. Non-cholera species can cause other human diseases.

V. vulnificus, opportunistically causes wound infections when an individual is exposed to contaminated water or swimming on marine water. Bacteria can disseminate to enter bloodstream and cause fulminant septicemia, however, this bacteria may primarily cause septicemia [134]. Mortality rate of septicemia with this bacteria reach 50%. Virulence factors of this bacteria includes, capsular polysaccharide, long chain LPS, siderophores (hyroxamate and vulnibactin), collagenase, metalloprotease and El Tor hemolysin.

V. alginolyticus, of low pathogenicity for human, causing superficial wound and ear infections. In a very rare occasion, these bacteria can cause septicemia. However, in co-infection with other bacteria it can cause very fatal septicemia especially among immunocompromised hosts [135].

V. parahemolyticus, this halophilic species produces thermostable hemolysin which lyses red blood cells and disrupts cell membrane cytoskeleton. On Wagatsuma's agar, they are beta hemolytic. This bacteria causes gastroenteritis which is characterized by abdominal pain, nausea, vomiting and diarrhea with or without blood in stool. Rarely, this bacteria can cause wound infections [9].

V. cholerae

This bacterium causes epidemic and pandemic cholera infections to humans. Strains of these bacteria are divided according to somatic O antigen (located on cell walls), as all serogroups have similar flagella H antigens. All pandemic strains were agglutinated by O1 antisera (mid 1930s) and further serotyped to three serogroups; Inaba, Ogawa and Hikojima. Epidemic strains O1 were further serotyped to two biotypes; Classical and El Tor (active hemolytic). El Tor was isolated in Egypt, El Tor Quarantine station. The biotype Classical was thought disappeared but Bangladesh reported its reemergence [135].

There are seven pandemic outbreaks of cholera in history. But in 1992, cholera-like illness emerged in India and rapidly spread to nearby eight countries (Pakistan, Bangladesh, Burma, China, Saudi Arabia, Nepal, Malaysia and Thailand). The causative serotype could not be identified similar to any of 138 existing serotypes therefore assigned O139 Bengal. The emergence of O139 Bengal suggested the beginning of eighth pandemic. Since then, cholera cases were caused by *V. cholerae* O1 biotype El Tor until in 2002 when O139 Bengal reemerged in India [136].

Pathogenesis and virulence factors of *V. cholera*

Induced gastroenteritis by *V. cholera* starts with attachment and penetration of these bacteria to gastric and intestinal mucosal epithelial cells. This takes place by the aid of flagella which facilitates motility and mucin which facilitates penetration. Then, bacteria release enterotoxin with two subunits, A (active) and B (binding). B subunits bind toxin molecules to G_{M1} ganglioside receptors specific to cholera toxins on intestinal epithelial cell membranes. On the other hand, one peptide (A1, toxic activity) of the A subunit catalyzes ADP-ribocylation of the Gs regulatory proteins. Gs activates adenylate cyclase which causes intracellular rise in cAMP preventing reabsorption of sodium ions across the brush-border membrane, increasing concentration of sodium, bicarbonate, potassium and chloride ions forcing water to be released into intestinal lumen from epithelial cells. Therefore resulting to accumulation of large amount of water, hence diarrhea manifest. If not managed early, can result to dehydration and electrolytes imbalance leading to hypokalemia, metabolic acidosis, shock and finally death [137].

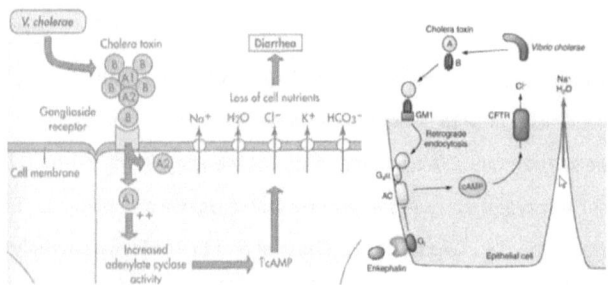

Figure 6: The mode of action of *V. cholera* toxin (Credit: Shomu's Biology)

Fastidious bacteria
Fastidious bacteria are slow growing (> 48 hours) and require complex nutritional requirements under specific culture conditions. They frequent gives false negative culture whenever their nutritional and culture conditions were not fulfilled. Which is clinically irrelevant? For that reason, bacteriologists should consider some other sensitive diagnostic methods such as molecular and immunological techniques. *Hemophillus, Neisseria, Campylobacter* and *Helicobacter* species are among most fastidious bacteria of medical importance to humans.

Helicobacter **species**

These fastidious gram negative spiral/curved bacteria producing catalase, oxidase and urease enzymes colonize gastrointestinal tracts of mammalian and avian. Intrinsic resistance to multiple antibiotics facilitated invention of selective culture media for these bacteria. Some selective supplements include Skirrow's supplement (contains: 5µg/ml trimethoprim, 10µg/ml vancomycin, 2.5 IU/ml polymixin B and amphotericin B) and Glaxo selective supplement A (GSSA). On 5% sheep blood agar supplement with either selective supplement, under 5-10%

CO^2 at 37⁰C for 2 to 5 days, the bacteria produces small translucent colonies. In tissue culture incubator, moist layers of absorbent gauze or a tray of distilled water should be placed at the bottom of culture plates to maintain humidity [138].

H. pylori

This bacterium asymptomatically colonizes more than 50% of people worldwide and majority acquires colonization during childhood. Acquisition of these bacteria happens via direct contact of person-to-person, or with vomitus and feces of infected/colonized person. These bacteria can change (by increase) the pH of its surroundings therefore effectively surviving acidity environment of the stomach. Most individuals are asymptomatically colonized, but these bacteria can become infectious and cause gastritis and peptic ulcers. Also, these bacteria have been linked with gastric and duodenal cancers. It was reported that, 50% and 80% of people with gastric ulcers and duodenal ulcers are infected with H. pylori. Moreover, 75% of people with mucosa associated lymphoid tissues (MALT) are infected with H. pylori. Infections with H. pylori stimulate inflammatory reactions, releasing neutrophils, eosinophils and dendritic cells. Furthermore, being intracellular bacteria of innate immune cells, H. pylori interferes phagosome maturation. To induce gastric adenocarcinoma, infection by H. pylori passes from gastritis to dysplasia through intestinal metaplasia and finally gastric cancer [139].

To achieve its pathogenesis, H. pylori possess different virulence factors. These factors are, flagella for adhesion and colonization of gastric and duodenal mucosa; urease enzyme to hydrolyze urea into ammonia and CO^2 whereby ammonia reduces gastric acidity to favor its environment; fibrillar adhesin for adhesion and colonization of mucosa; LPS, this endotoxin stimulates release of cytokines; leukocyte release and activating factors, this is a neutrophil activating protein; vacuolating cytotoxin (VacA), induces vacuole formation in eukaryotic cells; cytotoxin associated antigen (CagA), this antigenic protein promotes important response of tissue inflammation; and lastly is heat shock protein A and B (HspA and HspB) of unknown pathogenesis [140].

Campylobacter species

This Gram-negative curved/comma/S/C shaped bacteria are motile, catalase positive, oxidase positive and non-lactose fermenters are naturally colonizing poultry. Through eating of contaminated food, raw milk or contact with infected or colonized animal, humans acquires infections. This genus contains 17 species and 6 subspecies whereby *C. jejuni* and *C. coli* are common pathogens of humans. However, *C. fetus* a known causative agent of spontaneous abortion in sheep and cattle can also cause infection in humans. Growth of these species is favored at 42°C, 5-10% CO_2 for more than 48 hours. Increased temperature above 48°C destroys bacterial cells.

Pathogenesis and virulence factors of *Campylobacter* species

C. jejuni and *C. coli* are causative agents of gastroenteritis a condition known as campylobacteriosis which is characterized by diarrhea sometimes bloody diarrhea, fever, abdominal pain, headache and nausea with or without vomiting. Conditions may be fatal among very young children, elderly and immunocompromised especially people living with HIV/AIDS. Sometimes, bacteremia, bacterial hepatitis, pancreatitis and miscarriage are some of the reported complications of campylobacteriosis [141].

Campylobacter species have flagella for motility but for secretion of its invasive antigens known as Campylobacter invasive antigens (Cia) and cytolethal distending toxin which helps this bacteria to evade host immune system and induce host cells apoptosis which influence their limited time survival in the stomach [142]. Also, they produce cholera-like toxins, but its role in pathogenesis is not yet understood.

Hemophillus **species**

These Gram-negative pleomorphic small coccobacilli colonize upper respiratory tract, mouth, vagina and intestinal tract of man. They grow very well on chocolate agar because of its increased accessibility to growth factors required for their metabolic activities. These factors are factor X (hemin) and factor V (nicotinamide adenine dinucleotide, NAD). Requirements of growth factors vary among *Hemophillus* species, some requires only one factor while other requires both factors. Common species are *H. influenzae* (causative agent of neonatal sepsis and meningitis), *H. parainfluenzae*, *H. aegyptius*, *H. ducrey* (causative agent of chancroid), *H. hemolyticus* and *H. parahemolyticus* [143].

Table 2: *Hemophillus* species requirement of growth factors, X and V [143]

Hemophillus species	Factor V	Factor X
H. influenzae	√	√
H. parainfluenzae	√	×
H. ducrey	×	√
H. aegyptius	√	√
H. hemolyticus	√	√
H. parahemolyticus	√	×

Pathogenesis and virulence factors of *Hemophillus* species

H. Influenzae type b (Hib) is the common agent causing neonatal meningitis however it can cause septicemia, osteomyelitis, pneumonia and epiglottitis. Hib infections are most common among immunocompromised individuals especially with viral infections like HIV/AIDS. Through lymphatic drainage and/or septicemia, Hib reach meninges where they penetrate epithelium and endothelium layers without unknown mechanisms. But, Hib are virulent using fimbriae for adhesion; LPS and type b capsular polysaccharide for invasion; and protease (immunoglobulin A protease, IgAase) to evade host immune system and promotes its colonization. Conjugate Hib vaccine is available and very effective against Hib. However, less virulent, non-typable *H. influenzae*, commonly causing meningitis among adults [144].

H. ducrey is sexually transmitted, causing venereal chancroid disease known as genital ulcer disease (GUD) resembling syphilitic chancre but very painful and discharging ulcer with lymphadenitis. *H. ducrey* and HIV infections are known to facilitate one another. Odds ratio for HIV acquisition among individuals with H. ducrey infection ranges from 3 to 18 folds while for HIV seropositive individuals the odds ratio ranges from 10 to 100 folds. This happens because, ulcer provides easily and accessible portal of viral entry and viral shedding site. Virulence factors including pili, outer membrane proteins (OMPs), lipooligosaccharide (LOS), heat shock protein and iron regulating proteins facilitates *H. ducrey* pathogenesis. For effective treatment outcome, all sexual contacts should be traced and treated. Sometimes, treatment failure happen but very common among HIV seropositive individuals [145].

Neisseria species

These bacteria belong to the family *Neisseriaceae*. They are Gram-negative diplococci resembling coffee beans, catalase positive and oxidase positive. This genus, Neisseria was named after Germany bacteriologist who discovered it, Albert Neisser (1879). There are two important human causing diseases species; *N. gonorrhoeae* (gonococcus) causing gonorrhea and *N. meningitidis* (meningococcus) causing meningococcal meningitis and meningococcal septicemia. *N. meningitis* may colonize upper respiratory tract asymptomatically but it is never with *N. gonorrhoeae*. Gonorrhea disease has high prevalence but low mortality while meningococcal meningitis has low prevalence but high mortality. These bacteria are very sensitive towards drying and direct sunlight. Immediate culture is required in 5-10% CO_2 [146].

Neisseria gonorrhoeae

It is sexually acquired, affecting urethral mucosal membrane (in males) and mucosal membrane of endocervix (in females) causing gonorrhea. But, bacteria can disseminate to other tissues and cause prostatitis (in males), and ovaritis and salpingitis in females. *N. gonorrhoeae* is an intracellular pathogen found in polymorph-nuclear cells (neutrophils) of the gonorrhea exudates. Pathogenesis of this bacteria include pili for adhesion to mucosa membranes; lipooligosaccharide (LOS) endotoxins for formation of antiphagocytic vacuole to evade host immune response and protease (IgAase) which also for evading of host immune responses [146].

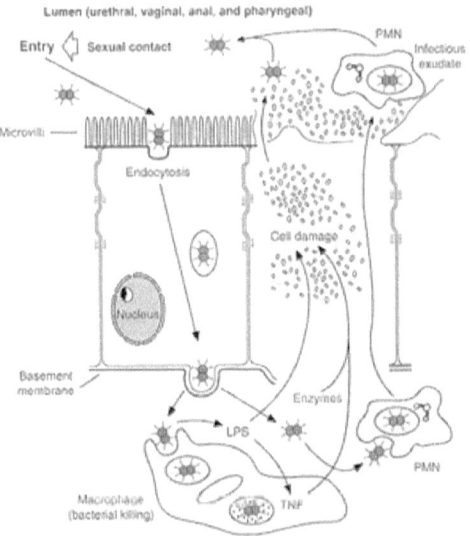

Figure 7: The pathogenesis of gonorrhea (Photo credit: Baron, Chapter 14)

Neisseria meningitidis

This bacterium is very similar to *N. gonorrhoeae* in staining and morphological characteristics. With its prominent its prominent antiphagocytic polysaccharide capsule, this bacteria is further grouped into 12 serogroups; A, B, C, H, I, K, L, X, Y, Z, 29E and W135. Disease causing serogroups (in humans) are A, B, C, Y and W135. This bacteria is very sensitive to temperature, all culture media should be pre-warmed to 37°C before inoculation. They should be incubated in 5-10% CO_2 at 37°C in a moist chamber [146].

Pathogenesis and virulence factors of *N. meningitidis*

When bacteria is aspirated into nasopharyngeal and oropharyngeal, it crosses mucosa barriers and enters bloodstream. In bloodstream it can cause mild symptoms of transient bacteremia (resolves in 1-2 days) to fulminant complicated meningitis disease with high mortality with 24 hours of hospitalization even with appropriate antibiotic therapy. Fulminant complicate meningitis is characterized with high grade fever, myalgias, nausea, vomiting, headache, restlessness, delirium and pulmonary insufficient. By using fimbriae, bacteria attach itself to mucosal membranes. To destroy and escape host immune responses, bacteria produces antiphagocytic polysaccharide capsule which prevents its phagocytosis and LOS endotoxin which suppress leukotriene B4 synthesis in leukocytes therefore deprives chemokinetic and chemotactic factors of leukocytes. This bacteria releases LOS endotoxin after death when it undergoes rapid autolysis [146]. This is the reason why mortality rate is very high even after administration of effective and appropriate antibiotic therapy.

Other Gram-negative bacteria of medical importance
Genus *Acinetobacter*

This diverse genus comprising Gram-negative bacteria that appear coccobacilli on non-selective agar but rods in liquid media. Generally, they are catalase positive, oxidase positive, utilizes citrate and showing twitching motility. This genus comprises more than 50 species which inhabits moist areas such as soil, water, sewage systems and most area of human skin. Among all, *A. baumannii* and *A. lwoffi* (occasionally causing meningitis) are frequently isolated from clinical specimens causing human infections.

Acinetobacter baumannii

Formerly known as *Herellea vaginicola*, *A. baumannii* causes opportunistic nosocomial infections especially among patients admitted in intensive care units (ICUs). However, community-acquired infections are now reported increasingly. Frequently nosocomial infections caused by *A. baumannii* are aspiration pneumonia (ventilator associated), bloodstream infections (BSIs) and urinary tract infections (UTIs). Other infections includes surgical site infections (SSIs), wound infections (WIs), endocarditis, burn infections and osteomyelitis [147]. Risk factors for acquisition of infections by *A. baumannii* are presence of indwelling invasive devices to patient such as urinary catheters and bloodstream catheters; prolonged hospital stay; open wounds; and contaminated inanimate hospital surfaces as reports of cross-transmission to patients exist.

Virulence factors of *A. baumannii* for its pathogenesis

For its effective pathogenesis, *A. baumannii* accommodates the following virulence factors; OmpA, lipopolysaccharide (LPS), capsular polysaccharide, phospholipase D, penicillin-binding protein, outer membrane vesicles, and acinetobactin mediated iron acquisition system. OmpA this mediates adherence and invasion of epithelial cells, biofilm formation, surface motility, serum resistance, induction of apoptosis in host cells. LPS conciliates dodging of the host immune response, triggering the host inflammatory response. Capsular polysaccharide moderates evasion of the host immune response, growth in serum. Phospholipase D arbitrates bacterial dissemination and serum resistance. Penicillin-binding protein mediates peptidoglycan biosynthesis, cellular stability, growth in serum. Outer membrane vesicles facilitate transfer of genetic material between bacterial cells and delivery of virulence factors to the cytoplasm of host cells. Acinetobactin mediated iron acquisition system for acquisition of iron needed for metabolism and causes cell apoptosis [148-151].

Antibiotics resistance among *A. baumannii*

Antibiotic resistance of *A. baumannii* to multiple or all antibiotics available has now become the global health threat. To the extent of resistance to antibiotics, some terminologies or definitions were proposed including multidrug resistant (MDR), extensive drug resistant (XDR) and pan drug resistant (PDR). MDR defined as resistance to at least three antibiotics in different classes. More than 80% of *A. baumannii* clinical isolates in ICUs are MDR [152-154]. XDR is defined as being MDR and resistant to carbapenems (doripenem, ertapenem, imipenem and meropenem). XDR-*A. baumannii* prevalence in ICUs reach as high as more than 40% [152-154]. PDR shall be defined as being XDR and also resistant to tigecycline and polymyxins (last-resort antibiotics) [155]. From different studies, prevalence of PDR-*A. baumannii* (resistant to colistin) ranges from 5% to 27.9% [156-158]. To achieve this high levels of resistance to multiple or all antibiotics, *A. baumannii* is equipped with multiple genes encoding antibiotics hydrolyzing enzymes and facilitating about modifications of antibiotics' target sites hence resistance to antibiotics. These genes are located either on bacterial core genome or on mobile genetic elements like transposon and plasmids. Bacteria produces aminoglycosides modifying enzymes, AMEs (*aph*A1, *aph*A6, *aac*C1, *aac*C2, *aad*B genes) to resist aminoglycosides; DNAgyrase (*gyr*A, *par*C genes) to resist quinolones; transposon mediated efflux pumps (*tet*B, *tet*M genes) to resist tetracyclines; extended spectrum beta-lactamases (CTX-M, SHV, TEM, VEB-1) to resist beta-lactam antibiotics expect carbapenems; carbapenemases and metallo beta-lactamases (KPC, VIM, IMP, SIM-1, OXA) to resist carbapenems; and modification of lipopolysaccharide by *mcr*-1 genes to resist polymyxins [155, 159, 160].

Genus *Pseudomonas*

Also known as *Pseudomonads*, are Gram-negative rods, catalase-positive, oxidase-positive, facultative anaerobes, hemolyse red blood cells, possesses one or more polar flagella which facilitates motility. They belong to the family *Pseudomonadaceae*. This genus comprises at least 191 species of which *P. aeruginosa* is known as opportunistic (primarily nosocomial) pathogen causing human infections [161].

P. aeruginosa

These environmental ubiquitous bacteria can resist high salt concentrations, substandard antiseptics or disinfectants and gives swimming-like movement in fluids using its single polar flagella. Nutritional requirements for these bacteria are as low as it can grow in distilled water. *P. aeruginosa* causes urinary tract infections (UTIs) bloodstream infections (BSIs), respiratory tract infections, skin and soft tissue infections, burn wound infections, osteomyelitis and arthritis. Also, *P. aeruginosa* produces pyoverdin (fluorescent) and pyocyanin (blue) pigments which gives the characteristic color of pus [161].

Pathogenesis and virulence factors of *P. aeruginosa*

This bacterium causes localized and systemic infections through adhesion (attachment), invasion and dissemination stages. Attachment to epithelial cells or mucosal membranes is facilitated by pili and protease enzymes which degrades mucosal barriers like fibronectin. Biofilm formation protects bacteria from host inflammatory responses and opsonization hence facilitates easy attachments. For invasion, bacteria use extracellular enzymes, elastases and alkaline protease. Elastases hydrolyze IgA, IgG, collagen, fibronectin and complements while alkaline protease lyses fibrin and interferes its formation. In addition, bacteria produce hemolysins, phospholipase to break lipids and lecithinase to break lecithin. By using pyochelin, a derivative of pyocyanin, bacteria acquires iron from surroundings for metabolism. These virulence factors, all together brings about dissemination to other tissues [161].

Acid fast bacilli (AFB)

AFB is Gram-stain variables rods comprised with cell walls containing mycolic acid and waxy. In 1882, Robert Koch stained tubercle bacilli by using hot solution of methylene blue for 24 hours. In the same year, Ehrlich used basic fuchsin and aniline oil as mordant, and then decolorized smears by using diluted mineral oil. Later on, Ziehl modified the later technique by using carbolic acid as mordant. In the same year, Rindfleisch, instead of using hot primary stain, he heated smears on the slides. In 1883, Neelsen combined basic fuchsin and carbolic acid (mordant) in a single solution [162].

Primary stain, basic carbol fuchsin (lipid soluble solution penetrates wax cell wall) penetrates cell walls into bacteria cells facilitated by steam heating of smears. Then, followed by decolorization using acid whereby, acid-fast bacilli resists decolorization and non-acid-fast bacilli become decolorized. The ability to resist decolorization "acid fastness", these bacteria was termed as "acid fast bacilli". Other acid fast staining techniques are classic and modified Ziehl-Neelsen stain, Auramine-rhadamine stain, Auramine-phenol stain and Kinyoun stain. Acid fast genera are *Mycobacterium*, *Nocardia* and *Actinomycetes* [162].

Genus *Mycobacterium*

This diverse genus belongs to the family *Mycobacteriaceae*. Its members differ in their in vitro growth requirements, reservoirs and modes of pathogenesis. Members of Mycobacterium are Gram-stain variable, slightly curved rods, aerobic, non-spore forming, and non-motile. These strictly pathogens (potential or opportunistic) of man are slow growing on bacteriological culture media requiring more than 1 week. Mycobacterium are divided into four major groups namely, *Mycobacterium tuberculosis* complex, *Mycobacterium ulcerans*, *Mycobacterium leprae* and nontuberculous Mycobacteria (NTM) [163, 164].

Mycobacterium leprae

This bacteria causes a chronic granulomatous disease of the skin, peripheral nervous system, eyes and mucosal membrane of the upper respiratory tract known as leprosy [165]. This bacteria multiplies very slow with an average of 5 years incubation period, however may range from 1 year to 20 years. In 2018 WHO reported 208619 new cases of leprosy globally [165]. Leprosy is categorized into paucibacillary, a mild form with low number of organisms causing infection and multibacillary, a multiple symmetric skin lesion and nodules with high number of infecting organisms. Routine bacteriological culture media cannot be used to isolate this bacteria, therefore diagnosis depends on clinical presentation and pathological findings [164, 166, 167]. Rifampicin and clofazimine, known as multidrug therapy (MDT) is recommended for treating of leprosy [165].

Mycobacterium ulcerans

This opportunistic pathogen of man causes ulcers (necrotizing skin disease) and osteomyelitis when people with bleached or bruised skin contact contaminated soil or water. However, mode of transmission is still unknown. This disease incubation period is 4.5 months ranging from 1 month to 9 months [168]. Ulcers caused by M. ulcerans are known as Buruli in Africa and Dairnsdale in Australia. Buruli ulcer is one among the 17 neglected tropical disease [169]. There were 2713 suspected new cases of Buruli ulcer disease in 2018, Nigeria, Australia and Ghana reporting most case [170]. It is difficult to isolate these bacteria by bacteriological culture media, therefore molecular based techniques are recommended for diagnosis. Surgical debridement and antimicrobial drugs (rifampicin and streptomycin) are recommended for treatment of this disease [171].

Mycobacterium tuberculosis complex (MTBC)

This is a group of closely related bacteria infecting humans and other mammals causing Tuberculosis (TB), they are bio-safety level III. Mycobacterium tuberculosis complex (MTBC) comprises of *M. tuberculosis*, *M. bovis*, *M. africanum*, *M. microti*, *M. pinnipedii*, *M. mungi* and *M. canettii*. TB causing organisms are transmitted through inhalation of aerosols and droplets containing organisms (tubercle bacilli). Organisms lodge in the lungs' alveoli whereby latent TB (in immune competent individuals) or active pulmonary TB (in immune compromised individuals) develops. TB causing pathogens can disseminate and infect other tissues leading to extra-pulmonary TB which contributes to 15-20% [172]. In 2017 WHO reported 10 million new cases of TB and 1.6 million deaths due to TB globally. About 558,000 among new cases in 2017, had rifampicin-resistant TB (RR-TB) of which 82% had multidrug resistant TB (MDR-TB). Of those with MDR-TB, 8.5% had extensive drug resistant TB (XDR-TB) [173]. Current TB treatment guideline consists four antibiotics, isoniazid (INH), rifampin (RIF), ethambutol (EMB) and pyrazinamide (PZA) for two months followed by INH and RIF for four months [174]. Patients' adherence is challenged with this long duration (6 months) of antibiotics therapy which consequently affect the effectiveness of treatment and further the emergency and spread of RR/MDR/XDR-TB [175].

Pathogenesis and virulence factors of MTBC

To cause TB, the pathogenesis of MTBC includes three major phases; transmission, surviving host immune and destruction of host tissues. To achieve it pathogenesis, MTBC uses the following virulence factors. Lipoarabinomannan (LAM) which inhibits the maturation of phagosome and triggers the release of cytokines (TNF-α, IL-6, IL-10 and IL-12), and induces apoptosis of macrophages. Lipomannan (LM), this is polymannosylated phosphatidylinositol mannoside (PIM), an antigen to innate immune system which activates macrophages and induces expression of cytokines (TNF-α, IL-8 and THP-1), also induces apoptosis of macrophages. Another virulence factor used by MTBC is trehalose 6,6'-dimycolate (TDM), this toxic lipid found in the mycobacteria cell walls inhibits acidification of phagolysosome, promotes angiogenesis and prevents calcium ions dependent phagosome-lysosome fusion therefore prevent killing of mycobacteria. Also, mycobacteria possess phthiocerol dimcocerosate (PDIM) and phenolic glycolipids (PGL) which facilitates resistant to detergents and protect mycobacteria from killing by reactive nitrogen intermediate species. Twin-argenite transporter (TAT transporter), this confers mycobacteria resistance to beta-lactam antibiotics [176, 177].

References
1. Debebe S: **Immunology and serology**. *Alemaya university, Ethiopia* 2004:1-17.
2. Schroeder Jr HW, Cavacini L: **Structure and function of immunoglobulins**. *Journal of Allergy and Clinical Immunology* 2010, **125**(2):S41-S52.
3. Britanica: **Antigen** In.
4. Janeway CA, Travers P, Walport M, Shlomchik M: **Immunobiology: the immune system in health and disease**, vol. 7: Current Biology London; 1996.
5. Forthal DN: **Functions of antibodies**. *Microbiology spectrum* 2014, **2**(4):1.
6. Aristizábal B, González Á: **Innate immune system**. In: *Autoimmunity: From Bench to Bedside [Internet]*. edn.: El Rosario University Press; 2013.
7. Riera Romo M, Pérez-Martínez D, Castillo Ferrer C: **Innate immunity in vertebrates: an overview**. *Immunology* 2016, **148**(2):125-139.
8. Juhn SK, Jung M K, Hoffman MD, Drew BR, Preciado DA, Sausen NJ, Jung TT, Kim BH, Park S-Y, Lin J: **The role of inflammatory mediators in the pathogenesis of otitis media and sequelae**. *Clinical and Experimental Otorhinolaryngology* 2008, **1**(3):117.

9. Greenwood D, Slack R, Peutherer J, Barer M: **Medical Microbiology A Guide to Microbial Infections**. *Churchill Livingstone, Edinburgh* 2007.
10. Abbas AK, Lichtman AH, Pillai S: **Cellular and molecular immunology E-book**: Elsevier Health Sciences; 2014.
11. **Bacterial Cell Wall Targets Identification** [https://www.creative-biolabs.com/drug-discovery/therapeutics/bacterial-cell-wall-targets-identification.htm]
12. Ingraham JL, Ingraham CA: **Introduction to microbiology: a case history approach**: Brooks/Cole; 2004.
13. Foster T: **Staphylococcus**. In: *Medical Microbiology 4th edition*. edn.: University of Texas Medical Branch at Galveston; 1996.
14. Pöhlmann-Dietze P, Ulrich M, Kiser KB, Döring G, Lee JC, Fournier J-M, Botzenhart K, Wolz C: **Adherence of Staphylococcus aureus to endothelial cells: influence of capsular polysaccharide, global regulatoragr, and bacterial growth phase**. *Infection and immunity* 2000, **68**(9):4865-4871.
15. Thammavongsa V, Kim HK, Missiakas D, Schneewind O: **Staphylococcal manipulation of host immune responses**. *Nature Reviews Microbiology* 2015, **13**(9):529.
16. Keener AB, Thurlow LT, Kang S, Spidale NA, Clarke SH, Cunnion KM, Tisch R, Richardson AR, Vilen BJ: **Staphylococcus aureus protein A disrupts immunity mediated by long-lived plasma cells**. *The Journal of Immunology* 2017, **198**(3):1263-1273.
17. Ross A, Shoff HW: **Toxic Shock Syndrome**. In: *StatPearls [Internet]*. edn.: StatPearls Publishing; 2018.
18. Korman NJ: **Macular, papular, vesiculobullous, and pustular diseases**. In: *Goldman's Cecil Medicine*. edn.: Elsevier; 2012: 2522-2532.
19. McAdow M, Missiakas DM, Schneewind O: **Staphylococcus aureus secretes coagulase and von Willebrand factor binding protein to modify the coagulation cascade and establish host infections**. *Journal of innate immunity* 2012, **4**(2):141-148.
20. Kateete DP, Kimani CN, Katabazi FA, Okeng A, Okee MS, Nanteza A, Joloba ML, Najjuka FC: **Identification of Staphylococcus aureus: DNase and Mannitol salt agar improve the efficiency of the tube coagulase test**. *Annals of clinical microbiology and antimicrobials* 2010, **9**(1):23.
21. Fisk A: **The technique of the coagulase test for staphylococci**. *British journal of experimental pathology* 1940, **21**(5):311.
22. Ehlers S, Merrill SA: **Staphylococcus saprophyticus**. 2018.
23. Zhou X, Li Y: **Atlas of Oral Microbiology: From Healthy Microflora to Disease**: Academic Press; 2015.
24. Patterson MJ: **Streptococcus**. In: *Medical Microbiology 4th edition*. edn.: University of Texas Medical Branch at Galveston; 1996.
25. Bryant AE, Stevens DL: **Streptococcus pyogenes**. In: *Mandell, Douglas, and Bennett's principles and practice of infectious diseases*. edn.: Elsevier; 2015: 2285-2299. e2284.
26. Terao Y: **The virulence factors and pathogenic mechanisms of Streptococcus pyogenes**. *Journal of Oral Biosciences* 2012, **54**(2):96-100.
27. Stevens D, Bryant A: **Group A streptococcus: virulence factors and pathogenic mechanisms**. *Available on www uptodate com, last updated* 2007, **13**:07-09.
28. **Virulence factors of Streptococcus pyogenes and their roles** [https://microbeonline.com/virulence-factors-streptococcus-pyogenes-roles/]

29. Dion CF, Ashurst JV: **Pneumonia, Streptococcus Pneumoniae**. In: *StatPearls [Internet]*. edn.: StatPearls Publishing; 2018.

30. **Streptococcus pneumoniae (pneumococcus): Overview** [https://www.news-medical.net/health/Streptococcus-pneumoniae-(pneumococcus)-Overview.aspx]

31. AlonsoDeVelasco E, Verheul A, Verhoef J, Snippe H: **Streptococcus pneumoniae: virulence factors, pathogenesis, and vaccines**. *Microbiol Mol Biol Rev* 1995, **59**(4):591-603.

32. Coykendall AL: **Classification and identification of the viridans streptococci**. *Clinical Microbiology Reviews* 1989, **2**(3):315-328.

33. Haslam DB, Geme JWS: **Viridans streptococci, Abiotrophia and Granulicatella species, and Streptococcus bovis**. In: *Principles and Practice of Pediatric Infectious Diseases*. edn.: Elsevier; 2012: 716-719. e711.

34. Upadhyaya PG, Ravikumar K, Umapathy B: **Review of virulence factors of enterococcus: an emerging nosocomial pathogen**. *Indian journal of medical microbiology* 2009, **27**(4):301.

35. Madsen KT, Skov MN, Gill S, Kemp M: **Virulence factors associated with Enterococcus faecalis infective endocarditis: a mini review**. *The open microbiology journal* 2017, **11**:1.

36. Hall-Stoodley L, Costerton JW, Stoodley P: **Bacterial biofilms: from the natural environment to infectious diseases**. *Nature reviews microbiology* 2004, **2**(2):95.

37. Winn WC: **Koneman's color atlas and textbook of diagnostic microbiology**: Lippincott williams & wilkins; 2006.

38. Gelfand MS: **Epidemiology and pathogenesis of Listeria monocytogenes infection**. *UpToDate (en línea)(consultado el 30/03/2016) Disponible en www uptodate com/contents/epidemiology-and-pathogenesis-of-listeria-monocytogenes-infection* 2012.

39. Rouquette C, Berche P: **The pathogenesis of infection by Listeria monocytogenes**. *Microbiologia (Madrid, Spain)* 1996, **12**(2):245-258.

40. Burkovski A: **Cell envelope of corynebacteria: structure and influence on pathogenicity**. *ISRN microbiology* 2013, **2013**.

41. Bernard K: **The genus Corynebacterium and other medically relevant coryneform-like bacteria**. *Journal of clinical microbiology* 2012, **50**(10):3152-3158.

42. Oliveira A, Oliveira LC, Aburjaile F, Benevides L, Tiwari S, Jamal SB, Silva A, Figueiredo HC, Ghosh P, Portela RW: **Insight of genus Corynebacterium: ascertaining the role of pathogenic and non-pathogenic species**. *Frontiers in microbiology* 2017, **8**:1937.

43. Spencer RC: **Bacillus anthracis**. *Journal of clinical pathology* 2003, **56**(3):182-187.

44. McDowell RH, Friedman H: **Bacillus cereus**. In: *StatPearls [Internet]*. edn.: StatPearls Publishing; 2018.

45. Walters PR, Zuckerbraun BS: **Clostridium difficile infection: clinical challenges and management strategies**. *Critical Care Nurse* 2014, **34**(4):24-33.

46. Ofosu A: **Clostridium difficile infection: a review of current and emerging therapies**. *Annals of gastroenterology: quarterly publication of the Hellenic Society of Gastroenterology* 2016, **29**(2):147.

47. Sun X, Savidge T, Feng H: **The enterotoxicity of Clostridium difficile toxins**. *Toxins* 2010, **2**(7):1848-1880.

48. Hassel B: **Tetanus: pathophysiology, treatment, and the possibility of using botulinum toxin against tetanus-induced rigidity and spasms**. *Toxins* 2013, **5**(1):73-83.

49. George EK, Vivekanandan R: **Clostridium Tetani.** In: *StatPearls [Internet].* edn.: StatPearls Publishing; 2018.
50. WHO: **Botulism.** In.; 2018.
51. Jeffery IA, Karim S: **Botulism.** In: *StatPearls [Internet].* edn.: StatPearls Publishing; 2017.
52. Uzal FA, Freedman JC, Shrestha A, Theoret JR, Garcia J, Awad MM, Adams V, Moore RJ, Rood JI, McClane BA: **Towards an understanding of the role of Clostridium perfringens toxins in human and animal disease.** *Future microbiology* 2014, **9**(3):361-377.
53. Birkhead G, Vogt R, Heun E, Snyder J, McClane B: **Characterization of an outbreak of Clostridium perfringens food poisoning by quantitative fecal culture and fecal enterotoxin measurement.** *Journal of clinical microbiology* 1988, **26**(3):471-474.
54. Sakaue M, Ota K, Nakamura E, Nitta M, Oka M, Oishi Y, Sano Y, Yonogi S, Takasu A: **Type A fulminant Clostridium perfringens sepsis indicated RBC/Hb discrepancy; a case report.** *BMC infectious diseases* 2019, **19**(1):1-3.
55. Stevens DL, Bryant AE: **The role of clostridial toxins in the pathogenesis of gas gangrene.** *Clinical Infectious Diseases* 2002, **35**(Supplement_1):S93-S100.
56. Hassan SA, Akhtar A, Khan M, Sheikh FN, Asghar H: **Frightening" Resistant Clostridial Myonecrosis: A Case Report.** *Cureus* 2019, **11**(4).
57. Petrillo TM, Beck-Sagué CM, Songer JG, Abramowsky C, Fortenberry JD, Meacham L, Dean AG, Lee H, Bueschel DM, Nesheim SR: **Enteritis necroticans (pigbel) in a diabetic child.** *New England Journal of Medicine* 2000, **342**(17):1250-1253.
58. Clarke LE, Diekmann-Guiroy B, McNamee W, Java DJ, Weiss SM: **Enteritis necroticans with midgut necrosis caused by Clostridium perfringens.** *Archives of Surgery* 1994, **129**(5):557-560.
59. Fafangel M, Učakar V, Vudrag M, Berce I, Kraigher A: **A Five Site Clostridium Perfringens Food-Borne Outbreak: A Retrospective Cohort Study/Izbruh Okužb S Clostridium Perfringens, Prenesenih S Hrano, Na Petih Lokacijah: Retrospektivna Kohortna Raziskava.** *Slovenian Journal of Public Health* 2015, **54**(1):51-57.
60. Kairys N, Garg M: **Gardnerella.** In: *StatPearls [Internet].* edn.: StatPearls Publishing; 2018.
61. Schwebke JR, Rivers C, Lee J: **Prevalence of Gardnerella vaginalis in male sexual partners of women with and without bacterial vaginosis.** *Sexually transmitted diseases* 2009, **36**(2):92-94.
62. Raj P: **Pathogenesis and laboratory diagnosis of Escherichia coli—associated enteritis.** *Clinical microbiology Newsletter* 1993, **15**(12):89-93.
63. Sánchez J, Holmgren J: **Virulence factors, pathogenesis and vaccine protection in cholera and ETEC diarrhea.** *Current opinion in immunology* 2005, **17**(4):388-398.
64. Wasey A, Salen P: **Escherichia Coli (E Coli 0157 H7).** In: *StatPearls [Internet].* edn.: StatPearls Publishing; 2019.
65. Raji M, Jiwa S, Minga M, Gwakisa P: **Escherichia coli 0157: H7 reservoir, transmission, diagnosis and the African situation: A review.** *East African medical journal* 2003, **80**(5):271-276.
66. Jenkins C, Chart H, Willshaw G, Cheasty T, Tompkins D: **Association of putative pathogenicity genes with adherence characteristics and fimbrial genotypes in typical enteroaggregative Escherichia coli from patients with and without diarrhoea in the United Kingdom.** *European Journal of Clinical Microbiology & Infectious Diseases* 2007, **26**(12):901-906.

67. Nataro JP, Steiner T, Guerrant RL: **Enteroaggregative Escherichia coli**. *Emerging infectious diseases* 1998, **4**(2):251.

68. Pabst WL, Altwegg M, Kind C, Mirjanic S, Hardegger D, Nadal D: **Prevalence of enteroaggregative Escherichia coli among children with and without diarrhea in Switzerland**. *Journal of clinical microbiology* 2003, **41**(6):2289-2293.

69. Terlizzi ME, Gribaudo G, Maffei ME: **UroPathogenic Escherichia coli (UPEC) infections: virulence factors, bladder responses, antibiotic, and non-antibiotic antimicrobial strategies**. *Frontiers in microbiology* 2017, **8**:1566.

70. Wurpel DJ, Beatson SA, Totsika M, Petty NK, Schembri MA: **Chaperone-usher fimbriae of Escherichia coli**. *PloS one* 2013, **8**(1):e52835.

71. Collinson S, Emödy L, Kay W: **Thin aggregative fimbriae from diarrheagenic Escherichia coli**. *Journal of bacteriology* 1992, **174**(13):4490-4495.

72. Spurbeck RR, Mobley HL: **Uropathogenic escherichia coli**. In: *Escherichia coli.* edn.: Elsevier; 2013: 275-304.

73. Russo TA, Davidson BA, Genagon SA, Warholic NM, MacDonald U, Pawlicki PD, Beanan JM, Olson R, Holm BA, Knight III PR: **E. coli virulence factor hemolysin induces neutrophil apoptosis and necrosis/lysis in vitro and necrosis/lysis and lung injury in a rat pneumonia model**. *American Journal of Physiology-Lung Cellular and Molecular Physiology* 2005, **289**(2):L207-L216.

74. Mills M, Meysick KC, O'Brien AD: **Cytotoxic necrotizing factor type 1 of uropathogenic Escherichia coli kills cultured human uroepithelial 5637 cells by an apoptotic mechanism**. *Infection and immunity* 2000, **68**(10):5869-5880.

75. Guyer DM, Radulovic S, Jones F-E, Mobley HL: **Sat, the secreted autotransporter toxin of uropathogenic Escherichia coli, is a vacuolating cytotoxin for bladder and kidney epithelial cells**. *Infection and immunity* 2002, **70**(8):4539-4546.

76. Agarwal J, Srivastava S, Singh M: **Pathogenomics of uropathogenic Escherichia coli**. *Indian journal of medical microbiology* 2012, **30**(2):141.

77. Drancourt M, Bollet C, Carta A, Rousselier P: **Phylogenetic analyses of Klebsiella species delineate Klebsiella and Raoultella gen. nov., with description of Raoultella ornithinolytica comb. nov., Raoultella terrigena comb. nov. and Raoultella planticola comb. nov**. *International journal of systematic and evolutionary microbiology* 2001, **51**(3):925-932.

78. Ashurst JV, Dawson A: **Klebsiella Pneumonia**. In: *StatPearls [Internet].* edn.: StatPearls Publishing; 2019.

79. Delcour AH: **Outer membrane permeability and antibiotic resistance**. *Biochimica et Biophysica Acta (BBA)-Proteins and Proteomics* 2009, **1794**(5):808-816.

80. Kumar A, Schweizer HP: **Bacterial resistance to antibiotics: active efflux and reduced uptake**. *Advanced drug delivery reviews* 2005, **57**(10):1486-1513.

81. Bansal S, Harjai K, Chhibber S: **Depolymerase improves gentamicin efficacy during Klebsiella pneumoniae induced murine infection**. *BMC infectious diseases* 2014, **14**(1):456.

82. Clegg S, Murphy CN: **Epidemiology and Virulence of Klebsiella pneumoniae**. *Microbiology spectrum* 2016, **4**(1).

83. Wang J-H, Liu Y-C, Lee SS-J, Yen M-Y, Chen Y-S, Wang J-H, Wann S-R, Lin H-H: **Primary liver abscess due to Klebsiella pneumoniae in Taiwan**. *Clinical Infectious Diseases* 1998, **26**(6):1434-1438.

84. Liu C, Guo J: **Hypervirulent Klebsiella pneumoniae (hypermucoviscous and aerobactin positive) infection over 6 years in the elderly in China: antimicrobial resistance patterns, molecular epidemiology and risk factor.** *Annals of clinical microbiology and antimicrobials* 2019, **18**(1):4.

85. Sánchez-López J, García-Caballero A, Navarro-San Francisco C, Quereda C, Ruiz-Garbajosa P, Navas E, Dronda F, Morosini MI, Cantón R, Diez-Aguilar M: **Hypermucoviscous Klebsiella pneumoniae: A challenge in community acquired infection.** *IDCases* 2019, **17**:e00547.

86. Shankar C, Nabarro LE, Anandan S, Ravi R, Babu P, Munusamy E, Jeyaseelan V, Rupali P, Verghese VP, Veeraraghavan B: **Extremely high mortality rates in patients with carbapenem-resistant, hypermucoviscous Klebsiella pneumoniae blood stream infections.** *J Assoc Phys India* 2018, **66**:13-16.

87. Arnold RS, Thom KA, Sharma S, Phillips M, Johnson JK, Morgan DJ: **Emergence of Klebsiella pneumoniae carbapenemase (KPC)-producing bacteria.** *Southern medical journal* 2011, **104**(1):40.

88. Robilotti E, Deresinski S: **Carbapenemase-producing Klebsiella pneumoniae.** *F1000prime reports* 2014, **6**.

89. Pitout JD, Nordmann P, Poirel L: **Carbapenemase-producing Klebsiella pneumoniae, a key pathogen set for global nosocomial dominance.** *Antimicrobial agents and chemotherapy* 2015, **59**(10):5873-5884.

90. Singh L, Cariappa M, Kaur M: **Klebsiella oxytoca: An emerging pathogen?** *Medical Journal Armed Forces India* 2016, **72**:S59-S61.

91. Darby A, Lertpiriyapong K, Sarkar U, Seneviratne U, Park DS, Gamazon ER, Batchelder C, Cheung C, Buckley EM, Taylor NS: **Cytotoxic and pathogenic properties of Klebsiella oxytoca isolated from laboratory animals.** *PloS one* 2014, **9**(7):e100542.

92. Herzog KA, Schneditz G, Leitner E, Feierl G, Hoffmann KM, Zollner-Schwetz I, Krause R, Gorkiewicz G, Zechner EL, Högenauer C: **Genotypes of Klebsiella oxytoca isolates from patients with nosocomial pneumonia are distinct from those of isolates from patients with antibiotic-associated hemorrhagic colitis.** *Journal of clinical microbiology* 2014, **52**(5):1607-1616.

93. Kang C-I, Kim S-H, Park WB, Lee K-D, Kim H-B, Oh M-d, Kim E-C, Choe K-W: **Bloodstream infections caused by Enterobacter species: predictors of 30-day mortality rate and impact of broad-spectrum cephalosporin resistance on outcome.** *Clinical infectious diseases* 2004, **39**(6):812-818.

94. Michalska A, Gospodarek E: **Enterobacter spp. bacteria-the taxonomy, characteristics, virulence factors and the methods for identification.** *POSTEPY MIKROBIOLOGII* 2007, **46**(1):39-47.

95. Jacoby GA: **AmpC β-lactamases.** *Clinical microbiology reviews* 2009, **22**(1):161-182.

96. Doijad S, Imirzalioglu C, Yao Y, Pati NB, Falgenhauer L, Hain T, Foesel BU, Abt B, Overmann J, Mirambo MM: **Enterobacter bugandensis sp. nov., isolated from neonatal blood.** *International journal of systematic and evolutionary microbiology* 2016, **66**(2):968-974.

97. Singh NK, Bezdan D, Sielaff AC, Wheeler K, Mason CE, Venkateswaran K: **Multi-drug resistant Enterobacter bugandensis species isolated from the International Space Station and comparative genomic analyses with human pathogenic strains.** *BMC microbiology* 2018, **18**(1):175.

98.   Pati NB, Doijad SP, Schultze T, Mannala GK, Yao Y, Jaiswal S, Ryan D, Suar M, Gwozdzinski K, Bunk B: **Enterobacter bugandensis: a novel enterobacterial species associated with severe clinical infection.** *Scientific reports* 2018, **8**(1):5392.
99.   Moehring R, Mahlen S: **Infections due to Serratia species.** *UpToDate Waltham, MA(accesat în Ianuarie 2015)* 2015.
100.   Khanna A, KhAnnA M, AggArWAl A: **Serratia marcescens-a rare opportunistic nosocomial pathogen and measures to limit its spread in hospitalized patients.** *Journal of clinical and diagnostic research: JCDR* 2013, **7**(2):243.
101.   Lin C-S, Horng J-T, Yang C-H, Tsai Y-H, Su L-H, Wei C-F, Chen C-C, Hsieh S-C, Lu C-C, Lai H-C: **RssAB-FlhDC-ShlBA as a major pathogenesis pathway in Serratia marcescens.** *Infection and immunity* 2010, **78**(11):4870-4881.
102.   Kurz CL, Chauvet S, Andrès E, Aurouze M, Vallet I, Michel GP, Uh M, Celli J, Filloux A, de Bentzmann S: **Virulence factors of the human opportunistic pathogen Serratia marcescens identified by in vivo screening.** *The EMBO journal* 2003, **22**(7):1451-1460.
103.   Jones RN, Baquero F, Privitera G, Inoue M, Wiedemann B: **Inducible β-lactamase-mediated resistance to third-generation cephalosporins.** *Clinical Microbiology and Infection* 1997, **3**:s7-s20.
104.   Ranjan K, Ranjan N: **Citrobacter: An emerging health care associated urinary pathogen.** *Urology annals* 2013, **5**(4):313.
105.   Sami H, Sultan A, Rizvi M, Khan F, Ahmad S, Shukla I, Khan HM: **Citrobacter as a uropathogen, its prevalence and antibiotics susceptibility pattern.** *CHRISMED Journal of Health and Research* 2017, **4**(1):23.
106.   Dzeing-Ella A, Szwebel T, Loubinoux J, Coignard S, Bouvet A, Le Jeunne C, Aslangul E: **Infective endocarditis due to Citrobacter koseri in an immunocompetent adult.** *Journal of clinical microbiology* 2009, **47**(12):4185-4186.
107.   Crawford SE, Daum RS: **Bacterial pneumonia, lung abscess, and empyema.** In: *Pediatric respiratory medicine.* edn.: Elsevier; 2008: 501-553.
108.   Hossain S, Wimalasena S, Heo G-J: **Virulence factors and antimicrobial resistance pattern of Citrobacter freundii isolated from healthy pet turtles and their environment.** *Asian J Ani Vet Adv* 2017, **12**:10-16.
109.   Harris P, Ferguson J: **Antibiotic therapy for inducible AmpC β-lactamase-producing Gram-negative bacilli: what are the alternatives to carbapenems, quinolones and aminoglycosides?** *International journal of antimicrobial agents* 2012, **40**(4):297-305.
110.   Janda J, Abbott S: **The genus Enterobacter.** *The Enterobacteria* 1998:148-177.
111.   Orrett FA: **Prevalence of Proteus species in urinary tract infections in a regional hospital in Trinidad.** *Zhonghua yi xue za zhi= Chinese medical journal; Free China ed* 1999, **62**(7):438-442.
112.   Szabo D, Paterson DL: **Proteus species.** *Antimicrobial therapy and vaccines* 2002, **1**:537-544.
113.   Armbruster CE, Mobley HL, Pearson MM: **Pathogenesis of Proteus mirabilis infection.** *EcoSal Plus* 2018, **8**(1).
114.   Ryan MP, O'Dwyer J, Adley CC: **Evaluation of the complex nomenclature of the clinically and veterinary significant pathogen Salmonella.** *BioMed research international* 2017, **2017**.
115.   Adley C, Ryan M: **The nature and extent of foodborne disease.** In: *Antimicrobial Food Packaging.* edn.: Elsevier; 2016: 1-10.

116. Salmon D, Smith T: **Report on swine plague.** *US Bur Anim Indus, 2nd Ann Rpt* 1885.
117. Microbiology SSotNCotlSf: **The genus salmonella lignieres, 1900.** *The Journal of hygiene* 1934, **34**(3):333.
118. Nataro JP, Bopp CA, Fields PI, Kaper JB, Strockbine NA: **Escherichia, shigella, and salmonella.** In: *Manual of Clinical Microbiology, 10th Edition.* edn.: American Society of Microbiology; 2011: 603-626.
119. Issenhuth-Jeanjean S, Roggentin P, Mikoleit M, Guibourdenche M, de Pinna E, Nair S, Fields PI, Weill F-X: **Supplement 2008–2010 (no. 48) to the White–Kauffmann–Le Minor scheme.** *Research in microbiology* 2014, **165**(7):526-530.
120. Ashurst JV, Woodbury B: **Salmonella Typhi.** In: *StatPearls [Internet].* edn.: StatPearls Publishing; 2018.
121. Soper GA: **The curious career of Typhoid Mary.** *Bulletin of the New York Academy of Medicine* 1939, **15**(10):698.
122. Manuel L FG, Ramos JM, Núñez A, Cuenca M, de Górgolas M: **Focal infections due to non-typhi Salmonella in patients with AIDS: report of 10 cases and review.** *Clinical infectious diseases* 1997, **25**(3):690-697.
123. Chen PL, Chang CM, Wu CJ, Ko NY, Lee NY, Lee HC, Shih HI, Lee CC, Wang RR, Ko WC: **Extraintestinal focal infections in adults with nontyphoid Salmonella bacteraemia: predisposing factors and clinical outcome.** *Journal of internal medicine* 2007, **261**(1):91-100.
124. Ibarra JA, Steele-Mortimer O: **Salmonella–the ultimate insider. Salmonella virulence factors that modulate intracellular survival.** *Cellular microbiology* 2009, **11**(11):1579-1586.
125. Magden ER, Mansfield KG, Simmons JH, Abee CR: **Nonhuman primates.** In: *Laboratory animal medicine.* edn.: Elsevier; 2015: 771-930.
126. Yabuuchi E: **Bacillus dysentericus (sic) 1897 was the first taxonomic rather than Bacillus dysenteriae 1898.** *International journal of systematic and evolutionary microbiology* 2002, **52**(3):1041-1041.
127. Ansaruzzaman M, Kibriya A, Rahman A, Neogi P, Faruque A, Rowe B, Albert MJ: **Detection of provisional serovars of Shigella dysenteriae and designation as S. dysenteriae serotypes 14 and 15.** *Journal of clinical microbiology* 1995, **33**(5):1423-1425.
128. Yang Z, Hu C, Chen J, Chen G, Liu Z: **A new serotype of Shigella boydii.** *Wei sheng wu xue bao= Acta microbiologica Sinica* 1990, **30**(4):284-295.
129. Chang Z, Zhang J, Ran L, Sun J, Liu F, Luo L, Zeng L, Wang L, Li Z, Yu H: **The changing epidemiology of bacillary dysentery and characteristics of antimicrobial resistance of Shigella isolated in China from 2004–2014.** *BMC infectious diseases* 2016, **16**(1):685.
130. Li Z, Wang L, Sun W, Hou X, Yang H, Sun L, Xu S, Sun Q, Zhang J, Song H: **Identifying high-risk areas of bacillary dysentery and associated meteorological factors in Wuhan, China.** *Scientific reports* 2013, **3**:3239.
131. Nie C, Li H, Yang L, Zhong G, Zhang L: **Socio-economic factors of bacillary dysentery based on spatial correlation analysis in Guangxi Province, China.** *PloS one* 2014, **9**(7):e102020.
132. Mattock E, Blocker AJ: **How do the virulence factors of Shigella work together to cause disease?** *Frontiers in cellular and infection microbiology* 2017, **7**:64.

133. Trucksis M, Michalski J, Deng YK, Kaper JB: **The Vibrio cholerae genome contains two unique circular chromosomes**. *Proceedings of the National Academy of Sciences* 1998, **95**(24):14464-14469.
134. Baker-Austin C, Oliver JD, Alam M, Ali A, Waldor MK, Qadri F, Martinez-Urtaza J: **Vibrio spp. infections**. *Nature Reviews Disease Primers* 2018, **4**(1):8.
135. Janda J, Powers C, Bryant R, Abbott S: **Current perspectives on the epidemiology and pathogenesis of clinically significant Vibrio spp**. *Clinical Microbiology Reviews* 1988, **1**(3):245-267.
136. Faruque SM, Chowdhury N, Kamruzzaman M, Ahmad QS, Faruque A, Salam MA, Ramamurthy T, Nair GB, Weintraub A, Sack DA: **Reemergence of epidemic Vibrio cholerae O139, Bangladesh**. *Emerging infectious diseases* 2003, **9**(9):1116.
137. Kaper JB, Morris JG, Levine MM: **Cholera**. *Clinical microbiology reviews* 1995, **8**(1):48-86.
138. Blanchard TG, Nedrud JG: **Laboratory maintenance of helicobacter species**. *Current protocols in microbiology* 2006(1):8B. 1.1-8B. 1.13.
139. Diaconu S, Predescu A, Moldoveanu A, Pop C, Fierbinţeanu-Braticevici C: **Helicobacter pylori infection: old and new**. *Journal of medicine and life* 2017, **10**(2):112.
140. Jemilohun AC, Otegbayo JA: **Helicobacter pylori infection: past, present and future**. *Pan African Medical Journal* 2016, **23**(1).
141. WHO: **Campylobacter**. In.; 2018.
142. Dasti JI, Tareen AM, Lugert R, Zautner AE, Groß U: **Campylobacter jejuni: a brief overview on pathogenicity-associated factors and disease-mediating mechanisms**. *International Journal of Medical Microbiology* 2010, **300**(4):205-211.
143. Tortora GJ, Funke BR, Case CL: **Microbiology: an introduction**: Pearson Higher Ed; 2015.
144. Musher DM: **Haemophilus species**. 1996.
145. Spinola SM, Bauer ME, Munson RS: **Immunopathogenesis of Haemophilus ducreyi infection (chancroid)**. *Infection and immunity* 2002, **70**(4):1667-1676.
146. Todar K: **Pathogenic Neisseriae: Gonorrhea, Neonatal Ophthalmia and Meningococcal Meningitis**. In.
147. Wong D, Nielsen TB, Bonomo RA, Pantapalangkoor P, Luna B, Spellberg B: **Clinical and pathophysiological overview of Acinetobacter infections: a century of challenges**. *Clinical microbiology reviews* 2017, **30**(1):409-447.
148. McConnell MJ, Actis L, Pachón J: **Acinetobacter baumannii: human infections, factors contributing to pathogenesis and animal models**. *FEMS microbiology reviews* 2013, **37**(2):130-155.
149. Russo TA, Luke NR, Beanan JM, Olson R, Sauberan SL, MacDonald U, Schultz LW, Umland TC, Campagnari AA: **The K1 capsular polysaccharide of Acinetobacter baumannii strain 307-0294 is a major virulence factor**. *Infection and immunity* 2010, **78**(9):3993-4000.
150. Gaddy JA, Tomaras AP, Actis LA: **The Acinetobacter baumannii 19606 OmpA protein plays a role in biofilm formation on abiotic surfaces and in the interaction of this pathogen with eukaryotic cells**. *Infection and immunity* 2009, **77**(8):3150-3160.
151. Luke NR, Sauberan SL, Russo TA, Beanan JM, Olson R, Loehfelm TW, Cox AD, Michael FS, Vinogradov EV, Campagnari AA: **Identification and characterization of a glycosyltransferase involved in Acinetobacter baumannii lipopolysaccharide core biosynthesis**. *Infection and immunity* 2010, **78**(5):2017-2023.
152. Nowak J, Zander E, Stefanik D, Higgins PG, Roca I, Vila J, McConnell M, Cisneros JM, Seifert H, WP4 MWG: **High incidence of pandrug-resistant Acinetobacter baumannii**

isolates collected from patients with ventilator-associated pneumonia in Greece, Italy and Spain as part of the MagicBullet clinical trial. *Journal of Antimicrobial Chemotherapy* 2017, **72**(12):3277-3282.

153. Banerjee T, Mishra A, Das A, Sharma S, Barman H, Yadav G: **High prevalence and endemicity of multidrug resistant Acinetobacter spp. in intensive care unit of a tertiary care Hospital, Varanasi, India.** *Journal of pathogens* 2018, **2018**.

154. Hatami R: **The frequency of multidrug-resistance and extensively drug-resistant Acinetobacter baumannii in west of Iran.** *Journal of Clinical Microbiology and Infectious Diseases* 2018, **2**(1).

155. Manchanda V, Sanchaita S, Singh N: **Multidrug resistant acinetobacter.** *Journal of global infectious diseases* 2010, **2**(3):291.

156. Abdulzahra AT, Khalil MA, Elkhatib WF: **First report of colistin resistance among carbapenem-resistant Acinetobacter baumannii isolates recovered from hospitalized patients in Egypt.** *New microbes and new infections* 2018, **26**:53-58.

157. Dobrewski R, Savov E, Bernards A, Van Den Barselaar M, Nordmann P, Van Den Broek P, Dijkshoorn L: **Genotypic diversity and antibiotic susceptibility of Acinetobacter baumannii isolates in a Bulgarian hospital.** *Clinical microbiology and infection* 2006, **12**(11):1135-1137.

158. Ko KS, Suh JY, Kwon KT, Jung S-I, Park K-H, Kang CI, Chung DR, Peck KR, Song J-H: **High rates of resistance to colistin and polymyxin B in subgroups of Acinetobacter baumannii isolates from Korea.** *Journal of Antimicrobial Chemotherapy* 2007, **60**(5):1163-1167.

159. Perez F, Hujer AM, Hujer KM, Decker BK, Rather PN, Bonomo RA: **Global challenge of multidrug-resistant Acinetobacter baumannii.** *Antimicrobial agents and chemotherapy* 2007, **51**(10):3471-3484.

160. Hsueh P-R, Teng L-J, Chen C-Y, Chen W-H, Ho S-W, Luh K-T: **Pandrug-resistant Acinetobacter baumannii causing nosocomial infections in a university hospital, Taiwan.** *Emerging infectious diseases* 2002, **8**(8):827.

161. Todar K: **Pseudomonas.** In.

162. Laboratoryinfo: **Ziehl-Neelsen Stain (ZN-Stain) : Principle, Procedure, Reporting and Modifications.** In.; 2019.

163. Pfyffer GE: **Mycobacterium: general characteristics, laboratory detection, and staining procedures.** In: *Manual of Clinical Microbiology, Eleventh Edition.* edn.: American Society of Microbiology; 2015: 536-569.

164. Forbes BA, Hall GS, Miller MB, Novak SM, Rowlinson M-C, Salfinger M, Somoskövi A, Warshauer DM, Wilson ML: **Practice guidelines for clinical microbiology laboratories: mycobacteria.** *Clinical microbiology reviews* 2018, **31**(2):e00038-00017.

165. WHO: **Leprosy.** In.; 2019.

166. mondiale de la Santé O, Organization WH: **Global leprosy update, 2015: time for action, accountability and inclusion.** *Weekly Epidemiological Record= Relevé épidémiologique hebdomadaire* 2016, **91**(35):405-416.

167. Cambau E, Chauffour-Nevejans A, Tejmar-Kolar L, Matsuoka M, Jarlier V: **Detection of antibiotic resistance in leprosy using GenoType LepraeDR, a novel ready-to-use molecular test.** *PLoS neglected tropical diseases* 2012, **6**(7):e1739.

168. WHO.

169. WHO: **Treatment of Mycobacterium ulcerans disease (Buruli Ulcer).** 2012.

170.   WHO: **Buruli ulcer (Mycobacterium ulcerans infection)**. 2019.

171.   Nienhuis WA, Stienstra Y, Thompson WA, Awuah PC, Abass KM, Tuah W, Awua-Boateng NY, Ampadu EO, Siegmund V, Schouten JP: **Antimicrobial treatment for early, limited Mycobacterium ulcerans infection: a randomised controlled trial**. *The Lancet* 2010, **375**(9715):664-672.

172.   Sinha P, Gupta A, Prakash P, Anupurba S, Tripathi R, Srivastava G: **Differentiation of Mycobacterium tuberculosis complex from non-tubercular mycobacteria by nested multiplex PCR targeting IS6110, MTP40 and 32kD alpha antigen encoding gene fragments**. *BMC infectious diseases* 2016, **16**(1):123.

173.   WHO: **END TB, Accelerator package** 2019.

174.   Organization WH: **Global tuberculosis report 2013**: World Health Organization; 2013.

175.   Caño-Muñiz S, Anthony R, Niemann S, Alffenaar J-WC: **New approaches and therapeutic options for Mycobacterium tuberculosis in a dormant state**. *Clinical microbiology reviews* 2018, **31**(1):e00060-00017.

176.   Forrellad MA, Klepp LI, Gioffré A, Sabio y Garcia J, Morbidoni HR, Santangelo MDLP, Cataldi AA, Bigi F: **Virulence factors of the Mycobacterium tuberculosis complex**. *Virulence* 2013, **4**(1):3-66.

177.   Echeverria-Valencia G, Flores-Villalva S, Espitia CI: **Virulence factors and pathogenicity of Mycobacterium**. *Mycobacterium-Research and Development Wellman Ribón, IntechOpen* 2018:231-255.

CHAPTER THREE

Antibiotics: overview, classification, mode of action and mechanisms of antibiotics resistance
The history of discovery of modern antibiotics era

Antibiotics are believed to exist before the discovery, development and release of true antibiotics. This was known as pre-antibiotic era. It was evidenced by scientist who found traces of tetracycline from skeletal remains of inhuman, the ancient of Sudanese Nuba who lived between 350-550 C.E [1].

Before the first discovery of true antibiotic, penicillin in 1928 by Alexander Fleming, a professor in Bacteriology, some scientists used other bacteria and molds to treat some bacterial infections (refer table below, adopted from Explorable) [2, 3].

Year	Origin	Description
1640	England	John Parkington in his book on Pharmacology recommended the use of molds in treatment.
1870	England	John Scott Burdon-Sanderson reported that covering of culture fluid with molds prevented growth of bacteria.
1871	England	Joseph Lister worked on human tissue with antibacterial action of what he called Penicillium glaucium on
1875	England	John Tyndall at the loyal society he explained antibacterial action of Penicillium fungus.
1877	France	Louis Pasteur explained that some bacteria may be used to kill other bacteria.
1897	France	Ernest Duchesne used Penicillium glaucium to heal infected guinea pigs.
1928	England	Alexander Fleming discovered the antibiotic substance called penicillin from Penicillium notatum.

Before the introduction of penicillin (pre-antibiotic era), it was difficult to treat people with bacterial infections such as rheumatic fever, pneumonia, gonorrhea or bloodstream infections. In hospitals, doctors could do was very little but only waiting and hoping for the best [3].

On 3 September, 1928, when returning from his holiday break, A. Fleming while sorting his petri dishes inoculated with bacteria Staphylococcus he observed that on one petri dish around the growth of contaminating mold, bacteria were clearly inhibited to grow. The contaminating mold were later identified as *Penicillium notatum* [3].

Later on, Fleming performed different experiments including extraction of "mold juice" which was capable of inhibiting growth of wide range of pathogenic bacteria including Streptococcus spp, Meningococcus and Diphtheria bacillus. He tried to purify the juice to pure penicillin but it found to be very unstable, therefore he kept using the crude juice. Its application was differentiation of penicillin sensitive from penicillin resistant bacteria [3].

Howard Florey and his colleagues at Oxford University, Sir William Dunn School of Pathology, worked on the purification and chemistry of penicillin. They turned penicillin from laboratory to life-saving antibiotic. Their work started in 1939, when movements of Second World War (WWII) were just beginning making their work very difficult. The team needed about 500 liters of mold filtrate (juice) a week for animal experiments and clinical trials, therefore to maximize production they used strange arrays of culture vessels including food tins, bedpans, milk churns and baths. Meanwhile, other biochemists (Norman Heatley and Edward Abraham) was working on extraction and purification of penicillin helping to step up production [3].

On 12 February, 1941, penicillin was first injected to human, Albert Alexander a 43 years old policeman who was developing a life-threatening infection affecting his eyes, face and lungs with huge abscesses. He made a remarkable recovery during the course of treatment however he died later from penicillin run out before the complete course of treatment. It was followed by better outcomes among other patients [3].

From then, different scientists, biochemists and companies such as Glaxo (now known as GlaxoSmithKline) and Kemball Bishop (now known as Pfizer) joined efforts in increasing the yield of penicillin [3].

Timeline of antibiotics discovery

From 1928 to 1987, different classes of antibiotics were discovered, developed and introduced to patient care. In between 1940 and 1960, this period is known as the "golden age of antibiotic discovery". Since 1987, the discovery, development and release of new antibiotic class were voided.

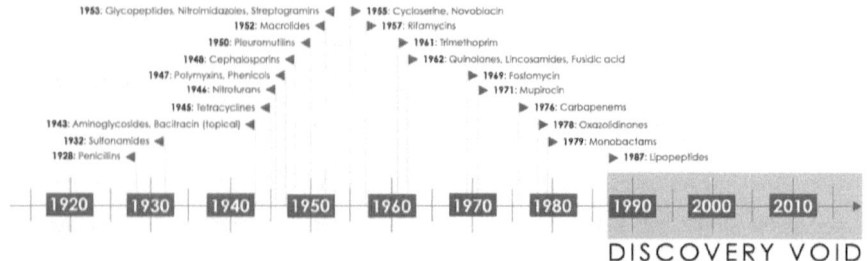

Figure 1: Timeline of antibiotics discovery, development and release (Source: ReAct, 2015).

The overview of antibiotics
Definitions

Antibiotic: is naturally occurring, synthesized or derivative of naturally occurring substances (or chemicals) which kill or inhibit growth hence multiplication of bacteria [4]. Antibiotic can be bactericidal or bacteriostatic [4].

Bactericidal antibiotics: are those antibiotics with ability of killing bacteria [5]. Examples of bactericidal antibiotics are penicillins, cephalosporins, glycopeptides, aminoglycosides, carbapenems and metronidazole [5]. However, effectiveness of bactericidal antibiotics is limited by infections which are deep seated or of poor blood supply where penetration of antibiotics become is reduced or poor. Also, during stationary phase of bacterial cell growth, bactericidal antibiotics are less effective. In the laboratory, during performing of antibiotic susceptibility testing, if heavy inoculum is inoculated on Muller Hinton agar (MHA) plate for susceptibility testing, bactericidal antibiotics may fail to achieve 100% effectiveness.

Bacteriostatic antibiotics: are those antibiotics which inhibit bacterial growth hence their multiplication [5]. Bacteriostatic agents hold bacteria at stationary phase of growth [6]. Examples of bacteriostatic antibiotics are macrolides, chloramphenicol, tetracycline, sulphonamides and trimethoprim [5]. However, when prescribed in combination, some of bacteriostatic antibiotics become bactericidal for example cotrimoxazole (a combination of trimethoprim and sulfamethoxazole). But sometimes, at higher dose, in single therapy, bacteriostatic antibiotics have shown bactericidal effects. Also, other bacteriostatic antibiotics, azithromycin, clarithromycin and erythromycin have shown bactericidal effects against susceptible cells of *S. pneumoniae* and *S. pyogenes* [6].

Bacteriostatic antibiotics has an advantage over bactericidal antibiotics, they inhibit protein synthesis therefore they are effective in diminish production of toxins (exotoxins and endotoxins) hence blocks mediators of host immune responses that results into clinical manifestations of a disease and sometimes fatal conditions [6].

Broad spectrum antibiotics: are those antibiotics with effectiveness against wide range of bacteria including both Gram-positive and negative bacteria [7]. Examples of broad spectrum antibiotics include tetracyclines, aminoglycosides, chloramphenicol and sulphonamides. However it is recommended to use broad spectrum antibiotics only when the implicating bacteria are not identified. If disease causing pathogen is identified it is recommended to use narrow spectrum antibiotics (as per antibiotics susceptibility patterns) to minimize emergence of multidrug resistant bacteria of the host's normal flora.

Antibiotics have selective toxicity nature which is selectively destroying bacteria cells without affecting host's cells. However whilst antagonizing bacterial cells causing disease they are also antagonizing the normal flora bacteria in or on hosts surfaces for example the useful normal bacteria in gastrointestinal tract. Also, long duration exposure to some antibiotics for example lincosamides (e.g., clindamycin) may results to secondary infections known as suprainfection for example pseudomembranous colitis [8].

Narrow spectrum antibiotics: are those antibiotics which are active against narrow range of bacteria, mostly one or few bacteria of either Gram-negative or positive bacteria [7]. Narrow spectrum antibiotics include glycopeptides (e.g., vancomycin).

Antibiotic resistance: inability of antibiotic to kill or inhibit growth (or multiplication) of bacteria at its optimal concentration. Resistance of bacteria to antibiotics may be of three kinds; intrinsic, circumstantial and/or acquired [9].

Intrinsic resistance: in this case, bacteria lack specific target (site of action) for antibiotic or presence of barriers to antibiotics reaching to their site of actions [9]. This is happening naturally. For example, impermeability of vancomycin antibiotic through outer membrane of

Gram-negative bacteria. Another example is, aerobic bacteria are naturally resistant against metronidazole (known antibiotic for treatment of aerobic bacterial infections) because aerobic bacteria fails to reduce metronidazole to its active form as they lack potential anaerobic mechanisms. Also, anaerobic bacteria are naturally resistant to aminoglycoside antibiotics as they lack oxidative metabolism for the uptake of these antibiotics.

Circumstantial resistance: in laboratory testing (in vitro), bacteria become susceptible to certain particular antibiotic of which become clinically (in vivo) resistant [9]. For example, first generation cephalosporins (1GCs) on in vitro laboratory testing are effective against bacteria isolated from cerebral spinal fluid causing meningitis but when administered to patient no recovery is observed. This is because, most of 1GCs are poor in crossing blood-brain barrier therefore they are not effective in treating of meningitis causing pathogens.

Acquired resistance: through different mechanisms bacteria become resistant to antibiotics it was once susceptible to [9]. This may happen from spontaneous chromosomal mutation due to antibiotics pressure or it can be acquired through acquisition of mobile genetic elements (MGEs) such as plasmids, insertion elements, transposons or chromosomal cassette (e.g., staphylococcal chromosomal cassette) harboring genes which produces enzymes that hydrolyzes different antibiotics making them ineffective against bacteria [10, 11].

Acquisition of MGEs is achieved through conjugation, transduction or transformation [10, 11]. Conjugation is an exchange of MGEs between bacteria cells through sex pili. When bacteriophage becomes the means of transportation of MGEs from one bacteria cell to another, this is known as transduction. While, a living bacteria picking up of free living MGEs such as free plasmid or from free genetic element from dying bacteria cell, this phenomenon is known as transformation. Therefore, if any of MGEs or free genetic element acquired has specific genes which produces significant enzymes that hydrolyzes antibiotics, changes bacteria trait from antibiotic susceptible to antibiotic resistant.

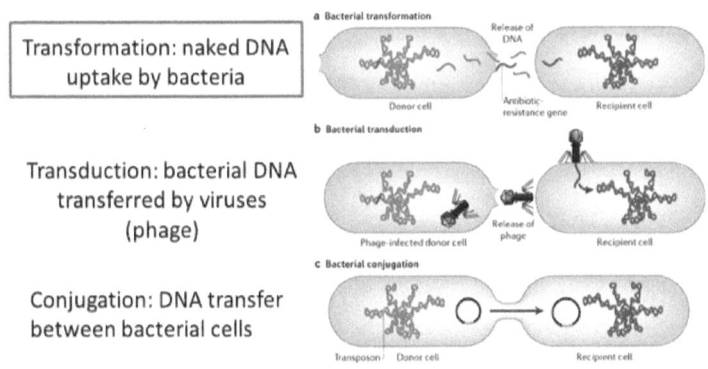

Transformation: naked DNA
uptake by bacteria

Transduction: bacterial DNA
transferred by viruses
(phage)

Conjugation: DNA transfer
between bacterial cells

Figure 2: Horizontal transfer of mobile genetic elements carrying genes which produces enzymes that has ability to hydrolyze antibiotics (Source: Nature Publishing Group, Nature review, 2016)

Clonal spreading

Clonal spreading is the propagation, establishment and spreading of a population of bacteria which is resistant to multiple antibiotics [12]. Briefly, once bacteria population comprises of very few cells (strains) which are resistant to multiple antibiotics. The majority of cells making this population are susceptible to almost all antibiotics. During this periodic time, bacterial infections are effectively treated by available antibiotics. Therefore, majority of susceptible cells will be killed (when exposed to antibiotics) leaving only resistant cells. This means, under selective pressure of antibiotics exposure, the majority of unfit cells (susceptible) will be selected out but the minority of fit (resistant) cells will be selected in. Then, selected in (very few) cells starts to propagate and re-establish to form a population of entirely resistant to multiple antibiotics for example multi-drug resistant (MDR) of extensive drug resistant (XDR) bacteria. Sometime a population resistant to all available antibiotics known as pa-drug resistant (PDR) bacteria [12]. These strains are then transmitted to locally (in hospital settings) and/or internationally (from continent to continent) via different vehicles. Locally, they are transmitted via colonization of humans or animals gastrointestinal tract (GIT) and contaminated hands of healthcare workers or inanimate surfaces or medical instruments. Internationally, they are carried in GITs of animals or humans migrating from one geographic boundary to another.

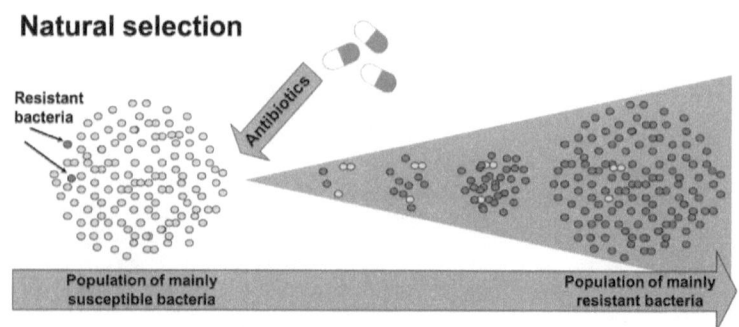

Figure 3: Clonal spreading of multiple resistant bacteria (Source: ReAct)

Classifications of antibiotics

Antibiotics are classified into different classes mainly based on their molecular structure, spectrum of activity, mode of action and route of administration [13]. However, antibiotics sharing molecular structure exerts the same patterns of toxicity and effectiveness [14]. Moreover, they are associated with the same kind of side effects. Based on molecular (chemical) structure, antibiotics are classified into beta-lactams, aminoglycosides, tetracyclines, macrolides, quinolones, sulphonamides, trimethoprim, oxazolidinones, glycopeptides and polymyxins [14].

Tetracyclines

Members of this class are sub-classified into first generation tetracyclines (e.g., chlorotetracycline, tetracycline, demeclocycline and oxytetracycline), second generation tetracyclines (e.g., doxycycline, lymecycline, minocycline, mecrocycline and methacycline) and third generation tetracyclines (e.g., tigecycline) [15]. Tetracycline was isolated from *Streptomyces* bacterium by Benjamin Duggar in 1945 [16]. But second generation tetracyclines are derivatives of semi-synthesis while third generation tetracyclines are total synthesis. All tetracyclines are associated with teeth discoloration among patients below 8 years of age [16].

Quinolones

Nalidixic acid was the first antibiotic to be discovered in this class, it was in early 1960s. It was accidentally discovered during researches on antimalarial drugs. Modification of quinolones basic structure led to introduction of new antibiotics with increased spectrum and efficacy [13,

17]. Other antibiotics in this class are floxacin, levofloxacin, ciprofloxacin, norfloxacin, temafloxacin, grepafloxacin, fravafloxacin and sparfloxacin. However, according to safety concerns, some antibiotics (e.g., grapefloxacin, sparfloxacin and temafloxacin) of this class were unregistered from clinical use [13, 17].

Polymyxins

This class contains antibiotics of polypeptides compound, polymyxins A-E, however only polymyxin B and polymyxin E (also known as colistin) are registered for clinical use in 1950s [18, 19]. Polymyxins were isolated from bacteria known as *Paenibacillus polymxa* subspecies *colistinus* [19]. Because of their nephrotoxicity and neurotoxicity effects, polymyxin antibiotics were once removed from clinical use in the early 1980s [18, 19]. Due to the emergence of extensive drug resistant (XDR) bacteria and pan-drug resistant (PDR) bacteria, polymyxin antibiotics were re-introduced for clinical use because of their effectiveness in treating infections with XDR and PDR bacteria [18, 19]. Frequently, *Acinetobacter baumannii* and *Pseudomonas aeruginosa* are clinically isolated as XDR and/or PDR. Therefore, they are reserved as "antibiotics of the last resort" [20].

Beta-lactams

Active molecule of beta-lactam antibiotics is a 3-carbon and 1-nitrogen ring which interferes synthesis of bacterial cell wall resulting to death or inhibited growth of the bacteria. Beta-lactam antibiotics include classes of penicillins, monobactams, cephalosporins and carbapenems.

Penicillins

Beta-lactam penicillin contains a nucleus known as aminopenicillanic acid ring. Most members of this class end with suffix –cillin which are penicillin G, penicillin V, nafcillin, oxacillin, amoxycillin, ampicillin, piperacillin, ticarcillin, mezlocillin and carbenicillin [21]. Among all antibiotics in this class and other classes of beta-lactams, penicillin G was the first discovered and introduced antibiotic by A. Fleming (1928) [21, 22]. It is a narrow spectrum, sensitive to *Streptococci, Meningococci* and *Treponema pallidum*. Due to high resistance of bacteria to antibiotics of this class, some penicillins are produced in a combination with penicillinase inhibitors. Penicillinase inhibitors are compounds which inhibit production of penicillinase enzymes from penicillin resistant bacteria. Examples of these antibiotics with penicillinase inhibitors are amoxycillin-clavulanic acid (also known as augmentin) and piperacillin-tazobactam [13].

Monobactams

This class contains only one antibiotic, azitreonam, a narrow spectrum, active against aerobic Gram-negative bacteria. Unlike other beta-lactam antibiotics, azitreonam comprises beta-lactam ring which is not fused to any other ring. Azitreonam was discovered and first reported by Sykes and his colleagues in 1981. It was isolated from bacteria known as *Chromobacterium violaseum* [13].

Cephalosporins

Cephalosporins were isolated from fungus known as *Cephalosporium acremonium* by Guiseppe Brolzu in 1945. Cephalosporins are bactericidal. Antibiotics in class cephalosporin are further sub-divided into 1st-5th generations (1GCs, 2GCs, 3GCs, 4GCs and 5GCs) depending on their target bacteria.

1GCs include cephalothin (oldest antibiotic of this generation), cefazolin (it is the only 1GC available in the USA), cephalexin, cephradrine, cefadroxil, cefonicid, ceforanide and cephaloridine [23, 24]. 1GCs are active against most of Gram-positive bacteria, moderate effective against Gram-negative bacteria and not effective against *Enterococci*, *Listeria* species, methicillin resistant *Staphylococci* and penicillin resistant *Pneumococci*.

2GCs are subgroup cephamycin (containing cefoxitin and cefotetan) and cefotiam, cefamandole, cefachlor, ceforanide and cefuroxime [25]. Generally, 2GCs are effective against both Gram-negative and Gram-positive bacteria. However they are not effective against *Pseudomonas* spp, *Enterococci*, *Acinetobacter* spp and *Bacteroides*. But subgroup cephamycin are effective against *Bacteroides* [25]. Subgroup cephamycin are quite stable to most of plasmid mediated beta lactamases though they are limited by chromosomal mediated cephalosporinases hence their application in screening of Amp C beta-lactamases production [25].

3GCs contain cefotaxime, ceftriaxone, ceftibuten, cefizox, cefdinir, ceftazidime, tazidime, cefoperazone and ceftizoxime [26]. Mostly, 3GCs have broad spectrum activity against Gram-negative bacteria however only ceftazidime and cefoperazone are the only antibiotics in this class that are effective against *Pseudomonas aeruginosa*. On the other hand, ceftizoxime and cefotaxime exerts the best activity against Gram-positive bacteria [26]. Generally, 3GCs are less effective towards beta-lactamases producing bacteria especially those producing inducible "chromosomal encoded" Amp C beta-lactamases. 3GCs are not recommended for prophylaxis use before surgery (however they are practically in use) due to emergence of multi-drug resistant bacteria colonizing patients and their association with super-infections or colonization particularly with *Enterococci* and *Candida* [27-29].

4GCs, structurally resembles 3GCs with only addition of a group of quaternary ammonium at C-3' position [30]. Cefpirome and cefepime are antibiotics making this generation [31]. Other members include cefoselis, cefozopran and cefclidine. They are less hydrolyzed by beta-lactamases including amp C beta-lactamase hence they have increased broad activity against Gram-negative bacteria including beta-lactamase producers [30, 31]. Moreover, cefpirome exhibit effective activity against Gram-positive bacteria such as penicillin resistant Pneumococci, Streptococcus viridans and methicillin susceptible Staphylococci [30]. These antibiotics are not effective against methicillin resistant Staphylococci and Bacteroides. 4GCs are less likely to induce resistance as compared to 3GCs because they penetrate bacterial cell walls very rapidly and they are hydrolyzed by beta-lactamases at a very low rate due to their low affinity towards these enzymes [30, 31].

5GCs, this generation include ceftobiprole, ceftaroline and ceftolozane. Ceftaroline is reported to have excellent activity against methicillin resistant *Staphylococci* while ceftobiprole has antipseudomonal activity [32]. Generally, 5GCs are less hydrolyzed by beta-lactamases however ceftolozane is combined with beta-lactamases inhibitor, tazobactam [33, 34].

Carbapenems

Carbapenems antibiotics were accidentally discovered during 1970s when researches were conducted to discover beta-lactamase inhibitors due to emergence of beta-lactamases producing bacteria that threatened the effectiveness of penicillins. Interestingly, thienamycin was discovered, it was isolated from bacteria known as *Streptomyces cattleya*. It was the first carbapenem discovered followed by commonly available and used now, imipenem, ertapenem doripenem and meropenem. Imipenem, a broad spectrum antibiotic exerts effective activity against aerobic and anaerobic bacteria; meropenem another broad spectrum antibiotic shows activity against Gram-negative bacteria; also ertapenem a broad spectrum antibiotic but it is limited to non-fermentative bacteria. Carbapenems are also known as "antibiotics of the last resort" because they are reserved for treatment of infections caused by multidrug resistant bacteria.

Oxazolidinones

This class comprises synthetic antibiotics which interferes bacterial synthesis of protein although their mechanism of action is not fully understood. Oxazolidinones antibiotics were approved for clinical use in 2000. Linezolid is an example of mostly used antibiotic in this class, which is a broad spectrum antibiotic effective against Gram-positive bacteria. Furthermore, linezolid is effective against methicillin resistant Staphylococci (e.g., MRSA), vancomycin resistant Pneumococci and anaerobic Gram-positive bacteria.

Aminoglycosides

These bactericidal antibiotics exert broad spectrum activity mainly towards Gram-negative bacteria but they also have coverage towards Gram-positive bacteria [35]. Examples of aminoglycosides are gentamicin, streptomycin, tobramycin, kanamycin, amikacin, netilmicin, debikacin, habekacin, paromomycin and neomycin [35-37]. Most members of this class are administered intravenously because they are polar compound hence poorly absorbed in the gastro-intestinal tract, however there are some which are taken orally (e.g., neofradin) and as eye drops (e.g., genoptic) [36, 37]. Aminoglycosides occurs naturally and some are semisynthetic derivatives (e.g., amikacin, habekacin, and dibekacin) [35].

Streptomycin was the first aminoglycoside to be discovered, it was isolated from *Streptomyces* [38]. All antibiotics of this class, aminoglycosides, ending with "mycin" were isolated directly or indirectly from this species [38]. But, those aminoglycosides ending with "micin" were isolated from *Micromonospora* species [38]. Streptomycin (the first aminoglycoside) was used for treatment of bubonic plague and tularemia [13]. It was found to be highly toxic hence the search for other alternatives of the same class, highly effective but less toxic, resulted to discoveries of other members [13, 39].

In most cases, aminoglycosides are reserved for treating of most serious infections caused by Gram-negative bacteria [39]. Aminoglycosides work synergistically with beta-lactam antibiotics [39]. In general, aminoglycosides are associated with ototoxicity and nephrotoxicity [39].

Sulphonamides

Antibiotics in this class are bacteriostatic exerting broad spectrum activity against Gram-positive and Gram-negative bacteria, but most of Gram-negative bacteria in the family *Enterobacteriaceae* shows resistance towards these antibiotics [40]. Moreover, sulphonamides have effect against cancerous cells [13, 41, 42]. Common members of this class are sulfamethoxazole, sulfadimethoxine and sulfadiazine [40]. At higher concentration or potentiated by combining with ormetoprim or trimethoprim they become bactericidal [40]. Generally, sulphonamides inhibit the synthesis of folic acid (essential for cell division) in bacteria [40]. Frequently reported side effects with sulphonamides use are mouth ulceration, nausea and hemolytic anemia [13]. Some literatures reported hypersensitivity reactions among patients who are allergic to sulfur-containing drugs, but this information and mechanism of reactions are still controversial [43, 44].

Trimethoprim

Trimethoprim is the common antibiotic in this class with a molecular structure of 2,4-diamino-5-(3',4'5'-trimethoxybenzyl)-pyrimidine [45]. Trimethoprim is the synthetic antibiotic, developed by Bushby and Hitchings purposely to potentiate sulphonamides as dihydrofolate reductase (essential enzyme for folic acid synthesis in bacteria cell) inhibitor however on its own it has antibacterial activity [45]. Trimethoprim has broad spectrum activity against aerobic Gram-positive and some Gram-negative bacteria [45]. Intrinsically, trimethoprim is not effective against *Pseudomonas aeruginosa*, *Treponema pallidum*, *Mycobacterium tuberculosis* and Bacteroides [45].

Commonly reported side effects of trimethoprim include nausea, diarrhea, rashes and itching [46]. Megaloblastic anemia, hyperkalemia, elevated serum creatinine, promoting production of shiga-like-toxin in entero-hemorrhagic Escherichia coli (EHEC) infections and risk of acute kidney injury are rarely reported side effects [47-50].

Macrolides

Structurally, this class contains macrocyclic lactose ring which is attached with one or more deoxy-sugars mostly cladinose and desosamine. Antibiotics in this class are bacteriostatic but at higher concentration they become bactericidal [46, 51]. Erythromycin was the first antibiotic to be discovered (in 1952), due to its adverse side effects mainly abdominal discomfort and cramps, nausea, vomiting and diarrhea, other antibiotics were discovered [46, 51]. Other antibiotics discovered include azithromycin, clarithromycin, fidaxomicin and roxithromycin which have few side effects. Generally, macrolides are administered to patients allergic to penicillins and cephalosporins, and as triple therapy in treatment of Helicobacter pylori infections [46, 51].

Glycopeptides

Vancomycin (isolated from *Amycolatopsis orientalis* in 1958) and teicoplanin (isolated from *Actinoplanes teichomyceticus* in 1978) are the only antibiotics of the first generation of this class which are registered for clinical use [52]. Naturally, glycopeptides contain cyclic peptide of 7 amino acids bounded with 2 sugars [53]. They exhibits broad spectrum activity against Gram-positive bacteria causing life-threatening infections such as methicillin resistant *Staphylococci* (MRSA) [53]. Therefore, they are known as "antibiotics of the last resort" [53]. Recently, bacteria resistant to glycopeptides (*Enterococci* and *Staphylococci*) has emerged, challenging for discovery researches of second generation glycopeptides [52, 53]. Second generation glycopeptides include telavancin (a derivative of vancomycin), dalbavancin (a derivative of teicoplanin-like-molecule) and oritavancin (a derivative of chloroeremomycin) are all semi-synthetic [53].

Lincosamides

Molecular structure of lincosamides contain pyrrolidine ring linked to a pyranose [54]. For clinical use, only lincomycin (natural isolated from *Streptomyces* species) and clindamycin (a semi-synthetic chlorinated derivative of lincomycin) are registered [55]. These antibiotics are bacteriostatic however at higher concentration they may be bactericidal [55]. Clindamycin is more active than lincomycin, effective against anaerobic bacteria [55]. Lincosamides (especially clindamycin) are associated with pseudomembranous colitis resulting from disruption of gastrointestinal flora [46].

Metronidazole

Metronidazole (also known as flagyl) was discovered (1959) and introduced for the treatment of *Trichomonas vaginalis*, but in 1962 it was first reported that, it has shown excellent activity against anaerobic bacteria after treating ulcerative gingivitis [56, 57]. Ten years later it was reported that, metronidazole was successful treated systemic anaerobic infections [56]. Currently, metronidazole is recommended for treatment of *C. difficile* infections, bacterial vaginosis caused by *Gardnerella vaginalis* and as triple therapy in treating of *H. pylori* infections [56].

Chloramphenicol

This antibiotic was discovered in 1947 from *Streptomyces venezuelae* however it is produced synthetically [58]. It exerts broad spectrum bacteriostatic activity against most of Gram-positive and negative bacteria [46]. However it is reported to have bactericidal effect against pathogens (especially *H. influenzae, S. pneumoniae* and *N. meningitidis*) causing meningitis due to its ability of forming high concentration in the cerebral spinal fluid (CSF) [58]. Its adverse side effects include aplastic anemia, bone marrow suppression, inhibit protein synthesis in mammalian mitochondria and it is toxic to neonates [46, 58, 59].

Selection of proper antibiotic therapy

The choice of proper antibiotic for treatment depends on factors such as culture (isolation of implicating bacteria) and susceptibility testing (susceptible antibiotics) and host factors including age, pregnancy conditions among female patients, history of adverse reactions, renal-hepatic function and site of infection. Antibiotics are toxic, their administration may present with no or mild to severe pharmacological side effects ranging from stomach upset to allergic reactions or birth defects (anomalies) or even death depending on age and condition of respective patient (e.g., neonate, pregnant or patient with renal failure). Therefore, selection of antibiotic to prescribe should be very cautious. For example, prescription of antibiotics during pregnancy considers the following categories, A, B, C, D and X, however sometimes unsafe antibiotics may be prescribed but when benefits outweighs risks.

Category A

These antibiotics present no possible harm to fetus because controlled studies in pregnant women demonstrated no risk to the fetus in the first trimester. Furthermore, there is no evidence of risk in later trimesters (second and third) [60]. Currently mycostatin is the only antibiotic listed under this category [61].

Category B

Based on animal studies, no risk demonstrated to fetus however no controlled studies in pregnant women [60]. Examples of antibiotics in this category are penicillins, cephalosporins (some have reported with increased risk of anomalies e.g., cephalexin, cefaclor and cephradrine), carbapenems, macrolides, aminoglycosides, clindamycin, azitreonam, nitrofurantoin (associated with hemolytic anemia at term) and metronidazole (shown evidence of carcinogenic in animals hence not recommended during first trimester) [62].

Category C

Studies on pregnant animal revealed adverse effects (abnormalities or death) on the fetus. There is neither controlled studies in both pregnant women and animals nor studies in pregnant women available [60]. Antibiotics under category C include carbapenem, fluoroquinolones, macrolides, aminoglycosides, sulfonamides, tetracycline, linezolid and trimethoprim [62]. In some circumstances, antibiotics under category C may be prescribed but only when potential benefits outweighs potential risk to fetus [60].

Category D

Antibiotics under this category have shown positive evidence of potential risk to fetus but under circumstances like life-threatening diseases and no safer alternative antibiotic is available or are not are available but not effective [60]. Examples of antibiotic in category D include tetracycline, oxytetracycline, naproxen and doxycycline [61].

Category X

Antibiotics under this category have shown clear evidence of fetal abnormalities based on human and animal studies [60]. Antibiotics of this category are not recommended to be used by women who are pregnant or planning to become pregnant because fetal risk outweighs any possible benefit [60]. Isotretinoin and thalidomide are antibiotics under category X [61].

Antibiotics combinations

- Antibiotics when used in combination, they exhibit additive, synergism or antagonist effect.
- Reasons for antibiotic combination
- Antibiotics are combined for the following purposes:
- Increased effectiveness hence prevent emergence of antimicrobial resistant bacteria
- For treatment of poly-microbial infections of different susceptibility patterns
- Initial therapy when causative bacteria agent is known yet identified and its susceptibility patterns is not known
- Combined antibiotic of less toxicity reduces toxic and side effects to patient
- Exerting additive or synergism effect therefore effective in treating bacterial infections

Antibiotics mode of action

Antibiotic agents target various sites on bacteria cell to achieve their bactericidal or bacteriostatic properties. These sites of antibiotics action include cell wall, cell membrane, ribosomes, cellular metabolism, and nucleic acids [63]. Their actions result into death or inhibition of growth of bacteria cell by inhibition of cell wall synthesis, disruption of cell membrane, inhibition of protein synthesis, inhibition of nucleic acid (DNA and RNA) synthesis, and metabolic pathways [63].

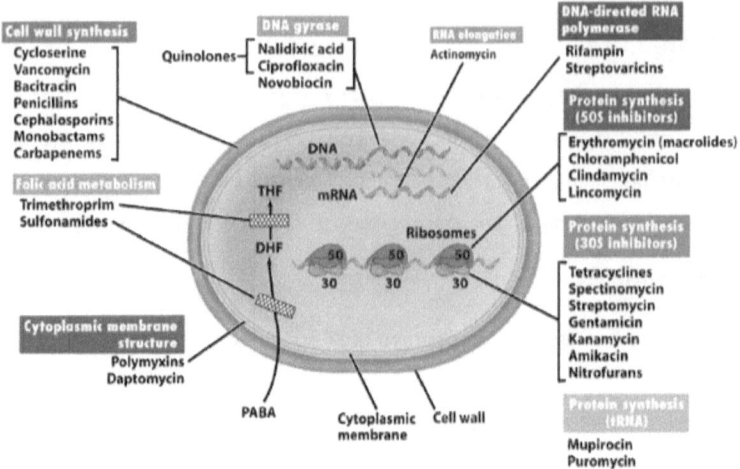

Figure 4: Sites of antibiotic targets in/on bacteria cell (source: Block Biology of Microorganisms 11/E, Pearson, 2016)

Inhibition of cell wall synthesis

Beta-lactam antibiotics; penicillins (ampicillin, amoxycillin, piperacillin), cephalosporins (first generation e.g., Cefazolin and cephalexin; second generation e.g., cefotetan, cefoxitin and cefuroxime and third generation e.g. ceftriaxone, cefotaxime and cefixime) and monobactams (azithromycin). Beta-lactam antibiotics acting by inhibiting the synthesis of bacterial cell wall are bactericidal. Briefly, synthesis of bacterial cell wall involves two major steps; transglycosylation and transpeptidation as explained previous. The final step of transpeptidation is the formation of peptidoglycan layer which is composed of repeating units of N-acetylglucuronic acid and N-acetylmuramic acid [64]. Then, the cross-linking of gaps between peptides (D-alanyl-D-alanine) attached on N-acetylmuramic acid is facilitated by peptidoglycan transpeptidase enzyme (found in bacterial cell membrane). Beta-lactam ring in beta-lactam containing antibiotics resembles D-alanyl-D-alanine therefore competitively acts on peptidoglycan transpeptidase enzyme as substrate. This enzymatic reaction is irreversible resulting to bacteriolysis and final cell death. In this case, beta-lactam containing antibiotics are termed as "suicide-inhibitors" [13, 64, 65].

In Gram-positive bacteria (e.g., *S. aureus*) cell wall formation involves transglycosylation (formation of linear monomers of sugar) and transpeptidation (interlinking of peptides to strengthen cell wall) processes. Binding of beta-lactam antibiotics on transpeptidation domain inhibit interlinking of peptides therefore a formation of weak cell wall which is easy to rapture and releasing of cytoplasmic contents hence cell death [13, 65].

Inhibition of protein synthesis

In bacteria, the core function of protein includes metabolic and physiological process, and structural composition. Therefore anything disrupting protein synthesis in bacteria may end up in death of the bacteria. Protein synthesis depends on information contained in deoxyribonucleic acid (DNA) which determines type and amount. Information in DNA is present in a form of genetic codes known as codons which is translated into messenger ribonucleic acid (m-RNA) under directives of DNA. Another similar biomolecule known as transfer-RNA (t-RNA) is also formed under directives of DNA. Both, m-RNA and t-RNA travels to ribosomes (in cytoplasm) which together with cytoplasmic factors, catalyzes the biosynthesis of protein. The t-RNA facilitates (at ribosomes) translation of codons in m-RNA to amino acids sequences the protein building blocks. Bacteria ribosome RNA (r-RNA) also known as 70S bacterial ribosome comprises two ribonucleoproteins, 30S (small subunit-SSU) and 50S (large subunit-LSU), possess 5S, 16S and 23S genes [13, 65].

Aminoglycosides and tetracyclines: inhibitors of 30S subunit

Aminoglycosides and tetracyclines are negatively charge hence they have affinity towards bacteria outer membrane which is negatively charged. Attachment of antibiotics from the two classes resulting into formation of large pores on outer membrane of bacteria hence facilitating their uptake into bacteria cytoplasm. In the bacteria cytoplasm, antibiotics are transported to ribosomes (site of action/target of action) by bacteria transport mechanism an active proton motive force which is energy dependent and oxygen requiring. In ribosomes, antibiotics interact with 16S r-RNA resulting to misleading and premature termination of m-RNA translation hence interfering with protein synthesis. The need of oxygen and active proton motive force to reach r-RNA, these antibiotics becomes less effective against anaerobic bacteria. Also, these antibiotics works synergistically with those antibiotics acting on bacterial cell walls (beta-lactam antibiotics such as penicillins, cephalosporins) [13, 65].

Chloramphenicol, lincosamides, oxazolidinones and macrolides: inhibitors of 50S subunit

These antibiotics interacts with 23S r-RNA of the 50S subunit preventing t-RNA from binding to A site of ribosome hence blocking the initial (translocation) or elongation (specifically macrolides and lincosamides) phases of protein synthesis [13, 65].

Inhibitors of nucleic acid synthesis

Quinolones interfere the function of helicase enzymes therefore preventing these enzymes from unwinding of double strand of DNA for DNA replication and repair. The binding of quinolones to helicase enzymes has high affinity therefore interfering it from unwinding and winding of DNA. In Gram-positive bacteria, quinolones targets RNA polymerase (topoisomerase IV) disrupting its activities hence preventing the synthesis of RNA. Quinolones has very low affinity towards mammalian RNA polymerase because, mammalian possesses topoisomerase II hence making them specifically antagonistic towards bacterial topoisomerase IV [13, 65].

Blocking of metabolic pathways

Sulphonamides and trimethoprim antibiotics resemble essential substrates needed for enzymes in metabolic pathways in bacteria. That, metabolic enzymes binds to these antibiotics instead of their normal substrates, therefore blocking key metabolic pathways in bacteria [13].

Breaking of bacteria cell membrane

Polymyxin antibiotics (colistin and polymyxin B) are cationic detergents which binds lipopolysaccharides on bacteria cell membrane. This binding disrupts lipid component and displaces magnesium and calcium resulting to increased permeability of the cell membrane. Consequently, osmotic gradient within the cell is affected therefore interfering nucleic acid synthesis and cellular metabolism [66].

Modern antibiotics era and post-antibiotics era

During the modern antibiotics era (from 1928), true antibiotics were discovered, developed and released for patients healthcare. During this period it was believed that bacterial infections were defeated because countless lives were saved. However a decade after first discovery and introduction of true antibiotic penicillin, its resistance was reported among *Staphylococcus* species [1].

Recently, antibiotics resistance among pathogenic bacteria mostly Gram-positive cocci and Gram-negative rods (*Acinetobacter baumannii*, *Pseudomonas aeruginosa* and family *Enterobacteriaceae*) has become global health concern. Bacteria are now resisting almost all available antibiotics including colistin the so called "antibiotic of the last resort". Following its re-introduction, colistin was reserved as the last bullet in treating of bacterial infections with multi-drug resistant, extensive drug resistant and pan-drug resistant bacteria.

In 2017, World Health Organization (WHO) published the first list of urgently needed antibiotics for the antibiotic resistant "priority pathogens" [67]. In the WHO catalogue, a list of antibiotic resistant "priority pathogens" comprises 12 families of bacteria with limited treatment options for human health [67]. Currently, bacteria resists large number of antibiotics including those reserved for treating of multi-drug resistant bugs. The WHO list grouped antibiotics resistant bacteria into three major "priority" groups namely priority 1; critical, priority 2; high and priority 3; medium.

Antibiotics resistant "priority pathogens" list in each group is follows as adopted from WHO, report of 2017;

Priority 1: CRITICAL

- Carbapenem-resistant *Acinetobacter baumannii*
- Carbapenem-resistant *Pseudomonas aeruginosa*
- Carbapenem-resistant and/or extended spectrum beta lactamase (ESBL) producing *Enterobacteriaceae*

Priority 2: HIGH

- Vancomycin-resistant *Enterococcus faecium*
- Methicillin-resistant and/or vancomycin intermediate and resistant *Staphylococcus aureus*
- Clarithromycin-resistant *Helicobacter pylori*

- Fluoroquinolone-resistant *Campylobacter* species
- Fluoroquinolone-resistant *Salmonella* species
- Cephalosporin-resistant and/or fluoroquinolone-resistant *Neisseria gonorrhoeae*

Priority 3: MEDIUM

- Penicillin-non-susceptible *Streptococcus pneumoniae*
- Ampicillin-resistant *Haemophillus influenzae*
- Fluoroquinolone-resistant *Shigella* species

Bacteria acquire antibiotics resistance through numbers of mechanisms but genome mutations and horizontal acquisition of mobile genetic elements are major mechanisms. Mobile genetic elements which may carry genes conferring antibiotics resistance includes; plasmids, insertion (IS) elements, transposons and phages.

New and effective antibiotics targeting this antibiotics resistant "priority pathogens" list are urgently needed. Any longer waiting will further this problem as previous reported that, by the end of 2050 if nothing will be done, about 300 million deaths and $100 trillion will be lost in the fight against antimicrobial resistance (AMR) [68]. Is this the sign of heading to post-antibiotics era as declared by CDC in 2013?

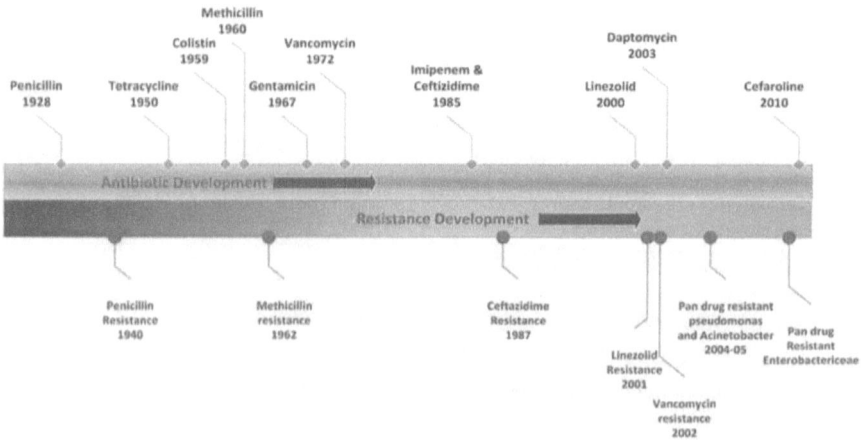

Figure 5: Timeline of emergence of antibiotics resistance (Source: IntechOpen, 2019)

The burden and impact of AMR is however still underestimated due to availability of limited information especially in most of low and middle income countries. Few available studies from low and middle income countries have reported very high magnitude of AMR infections with very few treatment options available, indirectly revealing high and serious impacts of AMR from these parts of the world. Availability of limited information from these countries is driven by many factors but the most important are; limited molecular diagnostic resources and unreliable phenotypic methods to detect AMR bacteria.

Mechanisms of antibiotics resistance
Resistance to beta-lactam antibiotics
Beta-lactamases

Mechanism of resistance of beta-lactam containing antibiotics is simply by bacterial production of beta-lactamase and/or penicillinase enzymes which hydrolyse the beta-lactam ring of an antibiotic (penicillins, cephalosporins, monobactams and carbapenems) [65, 69]. Production of these enzymes is encoded by genes which may be found on bacterial chromosome or cytoplasmic mobile genetic elements such as plasmids. In exposure to beta-lactam containing antibiotics, bacteria are induced to produce beta-lactamase enzymes. There are at least four classes of beta-lactamases: class A beta-lactamase, class B beta-lactamases, class C beta lactamases and class D beta-lactamases [65]. The commonest beta-lactamases classes are class A and C, at their active site (including class D), they are comprised with serine residues [70]. The metallo-beta-lactamases are comprised in class B beta-lactamase [70].

Class A beta-lactamases: these penicillinases known as extended spectrum beta-lactamases, ESBLs (CTX-M, TEM-1, and SHV-1) are found among bacteria in the family *Enterobacteriaceae*. Other ESBLs families though uncommon include PER-1, VEB-1, GES-1, GES-2 and IBC-2, they are mainly found in *Pseudomonas aeruginosa*. They are effective in hydrolyzing antibiotics in classes of penicillin, cephalosporins (1st, 2nd and 3rd generations) and monobactams. But they are not effective against methoxy-cephalosporins (e.g., cephamycins) and carbapenems. Also, they are inhibited by beta-lactamase inhibitors such as sulbactam, tazobactam and clavulanic acid [70].

Class B beta-lactamases: with addition to antibiotics hydrolyzed with ESBLs, metallo-beta-lactamases (e.g., New Delhi metallo-beta-lactamase) hydrolyzes carbapenems and they are not inhibited by beta-lactamase inhibitors [65].

Class C beta-lactamases: also known as cephalosporinases (e.g., Amp C beta-lactamase), they are able of hydrolyzing all beta-lactam antibiotics with exception to carbapenems. Contrarily to ESBLs, cephalosporinases are not inhibited by beta-lactamase inhibitors. There are two type of cephalosporinases, inducible and non-inducible. Inducible cephalosporinases are chromosomal encoded Amp C beta-lactamases produced by *Citrobacter freundii*, *Enterobacter cloacae*, *Serratia marcescens*, *Providencia stuartii* and *Morganella morganii*. Plasmid medicated (non-inducible) Amp C beta-lactamases are produced by other bacteria in the family Enterobacteriaceae such as *Salmonella* species, *Klebsiella* species and *Escherichia coli* [70, 71].

Class D beta-lactamases: also known as oxacillinases (OXA), they were described so, because of their effective hydrolysis of oxacillin however they are now able to hydrolyze a wide range of both narrow and broad spectrum beta-lactam antibiotics including penicillins, cephalosporins and even carbapenems. They were chromosomal encoded but now they are found among plasmids of diverse bacteria. Examples of oxacillinases are OXA-2, OXA-10 and OXA-23 (a carbapenem hydrolyzing class D beta lactamase (CHDL) also known as ARI-1). These enzymes are common among Acinetobacter baumannii and Pseudomonas aeruginosa and some bacteria of the family Enterobacteriaceae [72, 73].

Staphylococcal chromosomal cassette mec (SCCmec): Methicillin resistant *S. aureus* (MRSA) is any *S. aureus* with ability to hydrolyze beta-lactam antibiotics; penicillins, cephalosporins and monobactam making the antibiotics ineffective. Resistance among *S. aureus* is encoded by chromosomal gene, *mec*A which is carried within staphylococcal chromosomal cassette "SCC" *mec*, a mobile genetic element. SCC may be horizontally transferred between *Staphylococcus* species, however, recently have been reported among *Streptococcus pneumoniae*. SCC is recombined into host bacteria genome and inserted near origin of replication by using two recombinase genes; *ccr*A and *ccr*B which are also contained within it. The *mec*A gene in MRSA is responsible for production of "penicillin binding protein 2A" (PBP2A) reducing beta-lactam antibiotics affinity towards bacterial cell wall [74-76].

Resistance to aminoglycosides
Aminoglycosides modifying enzymes (AMEs)

Specifically bacteria mechanisms of resistance to aminoglycosides is achieved by aminoglycosides modifying enzymes (AMEs): phosphoryltransferases (APHs) encoded by *aph* genes, catalyzes ATP dependent phosphorylation of hydroxyl groups on aminoglycosides; adenylyltransferases (ANTs) encoded by *ant* genes, adenylating enzymes which add AMP from ATP donor to hydroxyl groups at 2",3",4',6 and 9 positions on aminoglycosides; and acetyltransferases (AACs) encoded by *aac* genes, acetylating enzymes of the amino groups found on aminoglycosides [77, 78]. Simply, AMEs hamper the binding of aminoglycosides to 30S ribosomal subunit [77].

16S r-RNA methyltransferases (RMTs)

Another mechanism of resistance to aminoglycosides is by production of RMTs, enzymes which modifies r-RNA nucleotide residues hence preventing aminoglycosides from binding to their site of action. RMTs are encoded by *arm*A, *rmt*B, *rmt*C, *rmt*D, *rmt*E, *rmt*F, *rmt*G and *rmt*H genes [77].

Inducible clindamycin resistance: clindamycin (class lincosamides) and erythromycin (class macrolides) antibiotics bind bacterial 23S component of the 50S ribosomal subunit. *Staphylococcus aureus* harboring *erm* gene encoding production of erythromycin inducible methylase enzyme confers bacterial resistance to both clindamycin and erythromycin antibiotics. When *S. aureus* harboring *erm* gene is exposed to erythromycin antibiotic it is induced to produce erythromycin inducible methylase which alters 23S component of the 50S subunit therefore inhibiting binding of clindamycin and erythromycin [79].

Resistance to chloramphenicol
Bacteria produces chloramphenicol transacetylase enzyme which modifies chloramphenicol by acetylating its hydroxyl groups making it unable to bind to ribosomal 50S subunit properly [65].

Other mechanisms of antibiotics resistance
Efflux pumps

There are five families of efflux pumps; ABC, RND (resistance-nodulation-division), MFS, SMR (small multidrug resistance) and MATE (multidrug and toxin extrusion). Genes encoding efflux pumps are either acquired or intrinsic. The *tet* genes of which about 22 have been identified to date, are acquired genes encoding efflux pumps which are harbored in the plasmids. Examples of intrinsic genes encoding for efflux pumps include *nor*A in *S. aureus*, *lmr*A in *Lactococcus lactis* and *acr*AB/*tol*C in *E. coli* [80].

The source of energy for ABC proteins is ATP but the other four proteins couple transport of substrate to ion gradient. Efflux pumps import or export only one specific substrate at a time however multidrug/polyspecific exporters are found in all the families suggesting polyspecific distributions. RND bridges inner and out membranes of bacteria cells of which single step is enough to export antibiotic from inside to outside of bacteria cell. Also, RDN and MFS are reported working synergistically resulting into increased minimum inhibitory concentration of tetracyclines [80].

Reduced permeability to antibiotics

Some bacteria (*Pseudomonas aeruginosa* and *Salmonella enterica*) on their cell walls they contains lipopolysaccharides (LPS) which consists lipid A and O-antigen. Bacteria with LPS moieties are intrinsically resistant to macrolides (erythromycin, azithromycin, clarithromycin) [81]. Also, other bacteria possess protein porin channels which allow entry of molecules of small molecular weight including antibiotics. When the expression or function of these porin channels is altered, entry of antibiotics into bacteria cells is reduced or inhibited [81].

Biofilm (resistance) formation and quorum sensing

Biofilm is a densely packed community of bacteria cells on surface (living or inert, moist or dry) and surround themselves with polymers (slime layer) [82]. It is estimated that 60-80% of pathogenic bacteria causing infections are also capable of forming biofilms [82, 83]. To form a biofilm, bacteria cells engage themselves into a quorum sensing (coordination mechanism or cell-cell communication via chemical vocabulary) [82, 84, 85]. Bacteria cell sense how many and at what distance are other cells located, then joining them and forming a biofilm. Quorum sensing takes place between the same and diverse bacteria species. To form a biofilm, number of genes are required for adhesion (e.g., *abp*A, *ssp*A/B, *bop*ABCD), quorum sensing (e.g., *com*X and *com*ABCDE), cell wall integrity (e.g., PBP2B, PBP5), metabolism (e.g., *ccp*A, *crc*) and stress response and antibiotics regulator (e.g., *dgk*) [84].

Polymer layer (slime layer) surrounding bacteria cells in a biofilm reduces permeability of modern antibiotics and natural antimicrobials of the host (for living things) [82]. Bacteria cells in a biofilm are up to 1000x more resistant to antibiotics than a free-living (planktonic) bacteria cell of the same strain [82, 84].

Causes and emergence of antibiotics resistance

The cause and emergence of antibiotic resistant bacteria (ARB) is multiple factors driven, mostly by inappropriate antibiotics use in hospitals, extensive antibiotics use in the community, extensive use of antibiotics in livestock husbandry and antibiotics discovery void [1].

Inappropriate antibiotic use in hospitals

About 50% of antibiotics are incorrectly or unnecessarily prescribed in hospitals [86]. Of which, up to 60% of unnecessarily (incorrectly) prescribed antibiotics are used in intensive care units (ICUs) [86, 87].

Extensive antibiotics use in the community

Mostly, in low and middle income countries antibiotics are easily and unregulated available over the counter [86]. Furthermore, they are sold at a very cheap prices without official prescription and sometimes they can be purchased online facilitating self and unprofessional medications [86].

Extensive antibiotics use in livestock husbandry

In livestock husbandry, antibiotics are extensively used as growth promoters resulting to emergence and colonization with ARB of these animals [86]. Humans acquire community infections or colonization with ABR from animals through shade off and consumption of animals' food products

Antibiotics discovery void

Pharmaceutical companies' efforts to discover new classes of antibiotics were discouraged by small investment of funds as reported that only $50 million was invested for antibiotics development as compared to $1 billion invested for neuromuscular drugs [86, 88]. It is reported that, 15 out of 18 largest pharmaceutical companies have abandoned the field of new antibiotics discoveries [86, 88].

References

1. Taneja N, Sethi S, Tahlan AK, Kumar Y: **Introductory Chapter: Stepping into the Post-Antibiotic Era—Challenges and Solutions**. In: *Antimicrobial Resistance-A Global Threat.* edn.: IntechOpen; 2019.
2. **History of antibiotics** [https://explorable.com/history-of-antibiotics]
3. **Discovery and development of penicillin** [http://www.acs.org/content/acs/en/education/whatischemistry/landmarks/flemingpenicillin.html]
4. McDonnell G, Russell AD: **Antiseptics and disinfectants: activity, action, and resistance**. *Clinical microbiology reviews* 1999, **12**(1):147-179.
5. Nemeth J, Oesch G, Kuster SP: **Bacteriostatic versus bactericidal antibiotics for patients with serious bacterial infections: systematic review and meta-analysis**. *Journal of Antimicrobial Chemotherapy* 2015, **70**(2):382-395.
6. Pankey G, Sabath L: **Clinical relevance of bacteriostatic versus bactericidal mechanisms of action in the treatment of Gram-positive bacterial infections**. *Clinical infectious diseases* 2004, **38**(6):864-870.
7. Maity A: **Antimicrobial Agents and its Ecological Effect**.
8. Chang T-W, Bartlett J, Gorbach S, Onderdonk A: **Clindamycin-induced enterocolitis in hamsters as a model of pseudomembranous colitis in patients**. *Infection and immunity* 1978, **20**(2):526-529.
9. Adekunle OO: **Mechanisms of antimicrobial resistance in bacteria, general approach**. *International Journal of Pharma Medicine and Biological Sciences* 2012, **1**(2):166-187.
10. Davison J: **Genetic exchange between bacteria in the environment**. *Plasmid* 1999, **42**(2):73-91.
11. McDaniel LD, Young E, Delaney J, Ruhnau F, Ritchie KB, Paul JH: **High frequency of horizontal gene transfer in the oceans**. *Science* 2010, **330**(6000):50-50.
12. **Antibiotic resistance** [http://www.columbia.edu/itc/hs/medical/pathophys/id/2009/antibresiNotes.pdf]
13. Etebu E, Arikekpar I: **Antibiotics: Classification and mechanisms of action with emphasis on molecular perspectives**. *Int J Appl Microbiol Biotechnol Res* 2016, **4**:90-101.
14. Ullah H, Ali S: **Classification of Anti-Bacterial Agents and Their Functions**. *Antibacterial Agents* 2017:1-16.
15. Chopra I, Roberts M: **Tetracycline antibiotics: mode of action, applications, molecular biology, and epidemiology of bacterial resistance**. *Microbiol Mol Biol Rev* 2001, **65**(2):232-260.

16. Sánchez AR, Rogers III RS, Sheridan PJ: **Tetracycline and other tetracycline-derivative staining of the teeth and oral cavity.** *International journal of dermatology* 2004, **43**(10):709-715.

17. Domagala JM: **Structure-activity and structure-side-effect relationships for the quinolone antibacterials.** *Journal of Antimicrobial Chemotherapy* 1994, **33**(4):685-706.

18. Falagas ME, Kasiakou SK, Saravolatz LD: **Colistin: the revival of polymyxins for the management of multidrug-resistant gram-negative bacterial infections.** *Clinical infectious diseases* 2005, **40**(9):1333-1341.

19. Gupta S, Govil D, Kakar PN, Prakash O, Arora D, Das S, Govil P, Malhotra A: **Colistin and polymyxin B: a re-emergence.** *Indian journal of critical care medicine: peer-reviewed, official publication of Indian Society of Critical Care Medicine* 2009, **13**(2):49.

20. Olaitan AO, Morand S, Rolain J-M: **Emergence of colistin-resistant bacteria in humans without colistin usage: a new worry and cause for vigilance.** In.: Elsevier; 2016.

21. Microbiology B: **Antimicrobial classification** 2016.

22. McGeer A, Fleming C, Green K, Low D: **Antimicrobial resistance in Ontario: are we making progress.** *Laboratory Proficiency Testing Program Newsletter* 2001, **293**:1-4.

23. Tartaglione TA, Polk RE: **Review of the new second-generation cephalosporins: cefonicid, ceforanide, and cefuroxime.** *Drug intelligence & clinical pharmacy* 1985, **19**(3):188-198.

24. Dumkiewicz R: **Potentiometric determination of cephalothin.** *Analyst* 1989, **114**(1):21-24.

25. Letourneau AR: **Learn how UpToDate can help you.**

26. Klein NC, Cunha BA: **Third-generation cephalosporins.** *The medical clinics of North America* 1995, **79**(4):705-719.

27. Geroulanos S, Marathias K, Kriaras J, Kadas B: **Cephalosporins in surgical prophylaxis.** *Journal of Chemotherapy* 2001, **13**(sup4):23-26.

28. Neu HC: **Third generation cephalosporins: safety profiles after 10 years of clinical use.** *The Journal of Clinical Pharmacology* 1990, **30**(5):396-403.

29. Dancer S: **The problem with cephalosporins** *Journal of Antimicrobial Chemotherapy* 2001, **48**(4):463-478.

30. Garau J, Wilson WW, Wood M, Carlet J: **Fourth-generation cephalosporins: a review of in vitro activity, pharmacokinetics, pharmacodynamics and clinical utility.** *Clinical Microbiology and Infection* 1997, **3**:s87-s101.

31. Giamarellou H: **Fourth generation cephalosporins in the antimicrobial chemotherapy of surgical infections.** *Journal of chemotherapy* 1999, **11**(6):486-493.

32. Takeda S, Nakai T, Wakai Y, Ikeda F, Hatano K: **In vitro and in vivo activities of a new cephalosporin, FR264205, against Pseudomonas aeruginosa.** *Antimicrobial agents and chemotherapy* 2007, **51**(3):826-830.

33. Zhanel GG, Chung P, Adam H, Zelenitsky S, Denisuik A, Schweizer F, Lagacé-Wiens PR, Rubinstein E, Gin AS, Walkty A: **Ceftolozane/tazobactam: a novel cephalosporin/β-lactamase inhibitor combination with activity against multidrug resistant gram-negative bacilli.** *Drugs* 2014, **74**(1):31-51.

34. Craig W, Andes D: **In vivo activities of ceftolozane, a new cephalosporin, with and without tazobactam against Pseudomonas aeruginosa and Enterobacteriaceae, including strains with extended-spectrum β-lactamases, in the thighs of neutropenic mice.** *Antimicrobial agents and chemotherapy* 2013, **57**(4):1577-1582.

35. Muraleedharan K, Avery M: In **Comprehensive Medicinal Chemistry II. Therapeutic Areas II: Cancer, Infectious Diseases, Inflammation, Immunology and Dermatology;** Taylor JB, Triggle DJ, Eds. In.: Elsevier: Amsterdam, The Netherlands; 2007.

36. Germovsek E, Barker CI, Sharland M: **What do I need to know about aminoglycoside antibiotics?** Archives of Disease in Childhood-Education and Practice 2017, **102**(2):89-93.

37. **What are aminoglycosides?** [https://www.everydayhealth.com/aminoglycosides/guide/]

38. Leggett JE: **Aminoglycosides.** In: Mandell, Douglas, and Bennett's principles and practice of infectious diseases. edn.: Elsevier; 2015: 310-321. e317.

39. Salvi RJ, Ding D, Eddins AC, McFadden SL, Henderson D: **Age, noise, and ototoxic agents.** In: Functional Neurobiology of Aging. edn.: Elsevier; 2001: 549-563.

40. Groman RP: **Miscellaneous Antibiotics.** In: Small Animal Critical Care Medicine. edn.: Elsevier; 2015: 944-949.

41. Sławiński J, Szafrański K, Vullo D, Supuran CT: **Carbonic anhydrase inhibitors. Synthesis of heterocyclic 4-substituted pyridine-3-sulfonamide derivatives and their inhibition of the human cytosolic isozymes I and II and transmembrane tumor-associated isozymes IX and XII.** European journal of medicinal chemistry 2013, **69**:701-710.

42. Xu F, Xu H, Wang X, Zhang L, Wen Q, Zhang Y, Xu W: **Discovery of N-(3-((7H-purin-6-yl) thio)-4-hydroxynaphthalen-1-yl)-sulfonamide derivatives as novel protein kinase and angiogenesis inhibitors for the treatment of cancer: Synthesis and biological evaluation. Part III.** Bioorganic & medicinal chemistry 2014, **22**(4):1487-1495.

43. Dibbern Jr DA, Montanaro A: **Allergies to sulfonamide antibiotics and sulfur-containing drugs.** Annals of Allergy, Asthma & Immunology 2008, **100**(2):91-101.

44. Carturan E, Basso C, Thiene G: **Molecular Pathobiology of Myocarditis.** In: Cellular and Molecular Pathobiology of Cardiovascular Disease. edn.: Elsevier; 2014: 135-159.

45. Masters BR: **Mandell, Douglas, and Bennett's Principles and Practice of Infectious Diseases, (2015) Eds: John E. Bennett, Raphael Dolin, Martin J. Blaser. ISBN: 13-978-1-4557-4801-3, Elsevier Saunders.** In.: Springer; 2016.

46. Cheesbrough M: **Medical Laboratory Practice in Tropical Countries, Part II.** In.: Cambridge University Press; 1984.

47. Crellin E, Mansfield KE, Leyrat C, Nitsch D, Douglas IJ, Root A, Williamson E, Smeeth L, Tomlinson LA: **Trimethoprim use for urinary tract infection and risk of adverse outcomes in older patients: cohort study.** bmj 2018, **360**:k341.

48. Naderer O, Nafziger AN, Bertino J: **Effects of moderate-dose versus high-dose trimethoprim on serum creatinine and creatinine clearance and adverse reactions.** Antimicrobial agents and chemotherapy 1997, **41**(11):2466-2470.

49. Choi MJ, Fernandez PC, Patnaik A, Coupaye-Gerard B, D'Andrea D, Szerlip H, Kleyman TR: **Trimethoprim-induced hyperkalemia in a patient with AIDS.** New england journal of medicine 1993, **328**(10):703-706.

50. Kimmitt PT, Harwood CR, Barer MR: **Toxin gene expression by shiga toxin-producing Escherichia coli: the role of antibiotics and the bacterial SOS response.** Emerging infectious diseases 2000, **6**(5):458.

51. **The appropriate use of macrolides** [https://bpac.org.nz/BPJ/2012/May/macrolides.aspx]

52. Kwun MJ, Hong H-J: **The activity of glycopeptide antibiotics against resistant bacteria correlates with their ability to induce the resistance system**. *Antimicrobial agents and chemotherapy* 2014, **58**(10):6306-6310.

53. Binda E, Marinelli F, Marcone GL: **Old and new glycopeptide antibiotics: action and resistance**. *Antibiotics* 2014, **3**(4):572-594.

54. Lincosamides, CID=56842237 [https://pubchem.ncbi.nlm.nih.gov/compound/56842237]

55. Spížek J, Řezanka T: **Lincosamides: chemical structure, biosynthesis, mechanism of action, resistance, and applications**. *Biochemical pharmacology* 2017, **133**:20-28.

56. Löfmark S, Edlund C, Nord CE: **Metronidazole is still the drug of choice for treatment of anaerobic infections**. *Clinical infectious diseases* 2010, **50**(Supplement_1):S16-S23.

57. Samuelson J: **Why metronidazole is active against both bacteria and parasites**. *Antimicrobial agents and chemotherapy* 1999, **43**(7):1533-1541.

58. Howard J, Balbi M: **Chloramphenicol-A review**. *Pediatrics in Review* 2004, **25**:284-288.

59. Tian F, Wang C, Tang M, Li J, Cheng X, Zhang S, Ji D, Huang Y, Li H: **The antibiotic chloramphenicol may be an effective new agent for inhibiting the growth of multiple myeloma**. *Oncotarget* 2016, **7**(32):51934.

60. **Antibiotics: Which Drugs Could Harm Your Unborn Baby?** [https://www.healthline.com/health/pregnancy/antibiotics-infections-during#1]

61. **Categories of Antibiotics** [https://www.babymed.com/medications/categories-of-antibiotics]

62. D P: **DRUGS IN PREGNANCY**. In.

63. Bbosa GS, Mwebaza N, Odda J, Kyegombe DB, Ntale M: **Antibiotics/antibacterial drug use, their marketing and promotion during the post-antibiotic golden age and their role in emergence of bacterial resistance**. *Health* 2014, **6**(05):410.

64. **Overview of beta-lactam antibacterials**

65. Kapoor G, Saigal S, Elongavan A: **Action and resistance mechanisms of antibiotics: A guide for clinicians**. *Journal of anaesthesiology, clinical pharmacology* 2017, **33**(3):300.

66. Long SS, Pickering LK, Prober CG: **Principles and practice of pediatric infectious disease**: Elsevier Health Sciences; 2012.

67. Organization WH: **WHO publishes list of bacteria for which new antibiotics are urgently needed**. *World Health Organization, Geneva, Switzerland* 2017.

68. King A: **Antibiotic resistance will kill 300 million people by 2050**. In.; 2014.

69. Drawz SM, Bonomo RA: **Three decades of β-lactamase inhibitors**. *Clinical microbiology reviews* 2010, **23**(1):160-201.

70. Jacoby GA, Munoz-Price LS: **The new β-lactamases**. *New England Journal of Medicine* 2005, **352**(4):380-391.

71. Mathers AJ, Peirano G, Pitout JD: **Escherichia coli ST131: the quintessential example of an international multiresistant high-risk clone**. In: *Advances in applied microbiology. Volume 90*, edn.: Elsevier; 2015: 109-154.

72. Antunes NT, Lamoureaux TL, Toth M, Stewart NK, Frase H, Vakulenko SB: **Class D β-lactamases: are they all carbapenemases?** *Antimicrobial agents and chemotherapy* 2014, **58**(4):2119-2125.

73. Antunes NT, Fisher JF: **Acquired class D β-lactamases**. *Antibiotics* 2014, **3**(3):398-434.

74. Wang L, Archer GL: **Roles of CcrA and CcrB in excision and integration of staphylococcal cassette chromosome mec, a Staphylococcus aureus genomic island.** *Journal of bacteriology* 2010, **192**(12):3204-3212.

75. Lowy FD: **Antimicrobial resistance: the example of Staphylococcus aureus.** *The Journal of clinical investigation* 2003, **111**(9):1265-1273.

76. Ito T, Kuwahara-Arai K, Katayama Y, Uehara Y, Han X, Kondo Y, Hiramatsu K: **Staphylococcal cassette chromosome mec (SCCmec) analysis of MRSA.** In: *Methicillin-Resistant Staphylococcus Aureus (MRSA) Protocols.* edn.: Springer; 2014: 131-148.

77. Krause KM, Serio AW, Kane TR, Connolly LE: **Aminoglycosides: an overview.** *Cold Spring Harbor perspectives in medicine* 2016, **6**(6):a027029.

78. **Mechanisms of Aminoglycoside Resistance** [http://www.uphs.upenn.edu/bugdrug/antibiotic_manual/aminoglycosideresistance.htm]

79. Leclercq R: **Mechanisms of resistance to macrolides and lincosamides: nature of the resistance elements and their clinical implications.** *Clinical Infectious Diseases* 2002, **34**(4):482-492.

80. Kaur P, Peterson E: **Antibiotic resistance mechanisms in bacteria: relationships between resistance determinants of antibiotic producers, environmental bacteria, and clinical pathogens.** *Frontiers in Microbiology* 2018, **9**:2928.

81. Abebe E, Tegegne B, Tibebu S: **A review on molecular mechanisms of bacterial resistance to antibiotics.** *EJAS* 2016, **8**(5):301-310.

82. **Biofilm bacteria** [https://mpkb.org/home/pathogenesis/microbiota/biofilm]

83. Lewis K: **Riddle of biofilm resistance.** *Antimicrobial agents and chemotherapy* 2001, **45**(4):999-1007.

84. Ali J, Rafiq QA, Ratcliffe E: **Antimicrobial resistance mechanisms and potential synthetic treatments.** *Future science OA* 2018, **4**(4):FSO290.

85. Higgins DA, Pomianek ME, Kraml CM, Taylor RK, Semmelhack MF, Bassler BL: **The major Vibrio cholerae autoinducer and its role in virulence factor production.** *Nature* 2007, **450**(7171):883.

86. Ventola CL: **The antibiotic resistance crisis: part 1: causes and threats.** *Pharmacy and therapeutics* 2015, **40**(4):277.

87. Luyt C-E, Bréchot N, Trouillet J-L, Chastre J: **Antibiotic stewardship in the intensive care unit.** *Critical care* 2014, **18**(5):480.

88. Bartlett JG, Gilbert DN, Spellberg B: **Seven ways to preserve the miracle of antibiotics.** *Clinical Infectious Diseases* 2013, **56**(10):1445-1450.

CHAPTER FOUR

Diagnostic Bacteriology
Introduction

Direct microscopic examination of smears (stained or unstained) from clinical specimens provide preliminary diagnostic results which guides further laboratory investigation procedures and initiation of empirical therapy while waiting for culture and sensitivity results. Staining reagents such as Gram-stain and Ziel-Nielsen stain, and culture media can be prepared in-house following standard guidelines. However, at each and every stage of reagents and culture media preparations, quality should be observed. Quality control ensures minimum laboratory errors hence provision of reliable laboratory results.

Basic stains in Bacteriology laboratory
Gram stain

It is a differential staining method of differentiating bacterial species into two large groups (Gram-positive and Gram-negative) based on the chemical and physical properties of their cell walls. The gram positive bacteria stains purple or blue due to the presence of crystal violet-iodine complex, and the gram negative bacteria stains pink or red due to the safranin or basic carbol fuchsin a counter-stain used [1, 2].

Some bacteria due to acidity of protoplasm have affinity to basic dye (react and hold firmly the basic dye crystal violet after treating with lugol's iodine), so they will appear blue or purple even if the decolorizer solution is applied; they termed as gram positive bacteria. Some bacteria will release the primary/basic stain after application of decolorizer and will take the color of secondary stain/counter stain and will appear pink/red; they termed as gram negative bacteria. The difference in dyes' affinity by bacteria cell wall is due to the thickness of peptidoglycan layer, the thicker layer much acidity hence affinity towards crystal violet and the thinner layer less acidity hence affinity towards carbol fuchsin [1, 2].

Materials and equipments

- Staining bacteria must be a pure 18 – 24 hours culture.
- Gram stains (crystal violet, lugol's iodine, 10% acetone in alcohol and 1:10 carbol fuchsin or safranin)
- Clean and greasy free glass slides

- Applicator sticks

- Sterile saline solution (0.85%)

- Oil immersion

- Microscope

- Known strains for quality control: *E. coli* ATCC 25922 and *S. aureus* ATCC 25923

Procedures for gram staining

- Prepare sample smear on clean, grease free glass slide and fix it by heat

- Flood the smear on glass slide with crystal violet (primary stain), 30-60 seconds

- Wash with clean running tape water

- Flood it with lugol's iodine; 30-60 seconds

- Wash with clean running tape water

- Decolorize until no color comes out (do not over or under decolorize)

- Wash with clean running tape water

- Flood it with neutral red (counter stain); 2-3 minutes

- Wash with clean running tape water

- Wipe/clean under slide with gauze, and then let it dry at room temperature

- Apply oil immersion, examine by 100X objective

- Report the result

Gram stain results interpretation

- Bacteria appearing as blue/purple to dark, violet in color after staining are GRAM POSITIVE

- Bacteria appearing as pink to red in color after staining are GRAM NEGATIVE

NOTE: Bacterial results interpretation under microscope MUST include color of staining (blue/purple are gram positive, pink/red are gram negative), arrangement (clusters, chains, pairs etc.) and morphology (cocci, bacilli).

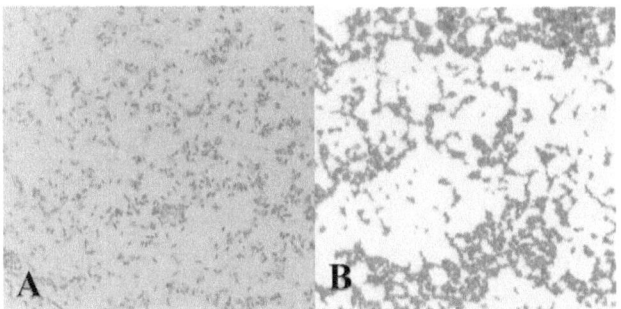

Figure 1; Gram stain (A). Gram negative rods bacteria. (B). Gram positive cocci in clusters.

Quality control of gram staining procedures and reagents

Controls must be run whenever staining schedule is taking place, to ensure appropriate staining procedures. And for every batch of new stain, controls must be run to ensure quality stains are made. Organisms used for quality control are *E. coli* (ATCC 25922), a gram negative rod (pink/red) and *S. aureus* (ATCC 25923), gram positive cocci (violet/purple)

Limitations of gram stains (causes of false positive and/or negative)
False gram negative may be due to:

- Cell wall damage due to antibiotic therapy
- Over de-colorization
- Too old lugol's iodine, not acts as mordant
- Smear from old culture

False gram positive may be due to:

- Too thick smear
- Under decolorization

Ziehl Nielsen (ZN) stains

Principle of the stain (hot technique)

ZN stain is used for staining acid fast bacilli (AFB). Acid fast bacilli includes; *Mycobacterium tuberculosis* a causative agent of tuberculosis, *Mycobacterium leprae* a causative agent of leprosy and *Norcadia asteroides* a causative agent of norcadiasis [3].

AFB has thick layer of mycolic acid and lipid in their cell walls, a waxy at room temperature. During staining procedure heat is applied to dissolves primary basic stain, strong carbol fuchsin into cell wall of the bacteria. AFB retains primary stain after application of the decolorize while other bacteria (normal flora of the upper respiratory tract) and background pick up the color of counter-stain, blue for methylene blue or green for methylene green. Acid fastness by AFB is due to retaining of basic stain, carbol fuchsin after application of decolorizer on mycolic acid of the cell walls [3].

Materials and equipments

- ZN stains (primary stain; strong carbol fuchsin, decolorizer; 20% sulphuric acid or 3% hydrochloric acid, counter-stain; methylene blue or methylene green)
- Clean and greasy free microscopic slides
- Sterile wire loop
- Source of heat
- Safety cabinet, level II
- Oil immersion
- Microscope

Procedures for ZN staining

- Make an oval smear (1 by 2 cm) on microscopic slide by using sterile wire loop
- Heat fix the smear on microscopic slide (four to six times passing over flame)
- Lie the slide on staining rack
- Flood the smear on slide with basic carbol fuchsin
- Apply heat (flame) under the smear on slide till steam comes out, do not boil
- After steam comes out, remove source of flame and wait for 5 minutes
- Then wash with running tap water, hold tilt the slide
- Decolorize by using available decolorizer till no primary color comes out the stained smear
- Apply counter-stain dye for 10 minutes
- Wash smear by using running tap water, and tilt the slide to air dry
- Examine under oil immersion objective

Results interpretation of ZN stain

AFB will stain red against the bluish or greenish background and other normal flora of the upper respiratory tract. AFB will be seen as short rods and *Norcadia* spp will be seen as long, thin and filamentous.

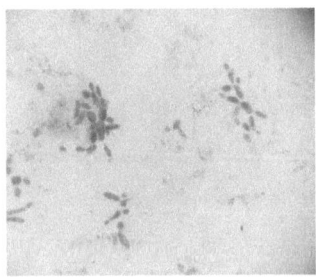

Figure 2; ZN stained smear from immunocompromised patients showing reddish rods (AFB), against bluish background and bluish budding yeast cells.

Reporting and grading of AFB under microscope[4].

Negative; no AFB seen (0 AFB/100 fields)

Scanty; 1-9 AFB/100 fields (report actual number)

Plus one (+1); 10-99 AFB/100 fields

Plus two (+2); 1-10 AFB/fields in 50 fields

Plus three (+3); '10 AFB/field in 20 fields

Modified ZN stain

Modified ZN stain was established for identification of *Mycobacterium tuberculosis* causing extra-pulmonary tuberculosis in cerebral spinal fluid (CSF) and exudate specimens. This technique can also be employed to examine coccidian protozoa of *Cryptosporidium* spp, *Isospora belli* and *Cyclospora* spp oocysts which cannot be well identified by concentration technique in stool specimens [5-8].

Materials and equipments

- Falcon tubes

- Wooden applicator sticks
- Clean greasy free microscopic glass slides
- 10% formalin
- Ethyl acetate
- Pasteur pipettes
- Centrifuge machine
- Light microscope

Concentration technique for stool specimens for modified ZN staining [9].

- Sieve stool specimen thoroughly through clean absorbent gauze into falcon tube
- Clean water or normal saline can be used to adjust volume
- Centrifuge stool sample for 1 minute at 500 revolution per minute (rpm)
- Discard supernatant, and mix well pellets
- Add 10% formalin in tube containing stool pellets and mix well (volume; 1 part of stool pellets and 10 parts of 10% formalin)
- Add ethyl acetate into tube containing a mixture of stool pellets and 10% formalin and mix well (volume; 2 parts of ethyl acetate and 5 parts mixture of stool pellets and 10% formalin)
- Centrifuge the above mixture at 500 rpm for 1 minute, discards three layers of supernants and use the pellets for making smears for modified ZN staining technique

Note: for identification of *Mycobacterium tuberculosis* in CSF and exudate specimens, concentration of specimens is only by centrifugation. Sediments or pellets are then used for making smears to be stained by modified ZN stain.

Staining procedures for modified ZN stain

- After making smears, allow to complete air dry
- Fix in absolute methanol for 3 to 5 minutes
- Stain with strong carbol fuchsin for 10 to 15 minutes
- Thoroughly rinse with running tap water
- Decolorize by using 1% acid alcohol (hydrochloric acid (HCL) in methanol) for 15 seconds

- Rinse thoroughly with running tap water
- Counter-stain with 3% methylene blue or 0.4% malachite green for 30 seconds
- Rinse thoroughly with running tap water and allow to air dry
- Examine under microscope by using oil immersion objective lens

Modified ZN stain results interpretation

Under microscope, species of *Mycobacterium tuberculosis*, *Cryptosporidium parvum*, *Isospora belli* and *Cyclospora* oocysts are red stained against bluish (if methylene blue is used) or greenish (if malachite green is used) background.

Preparation of stains and reagents
Crystal violet (primary gram stain dye)

Materials are crystal violet powder, ammonium oxalate, absolute alcohol (methanol or ethanol) and distilled water. Mix the mentioned material as follows; 10 gram of crystal violet powder, 4.5 gram of ammonium oxalate, 47.5 ml of absolute ethanol and 438 ml of distilled water to sum up to 500 ml of crystal violet stain dye.

Lugol's iodine (mordant)

Potassium iodide powder, iodine crystals and distilled water are the materials for making Lugol's iodine mordant. These materials are mixed in the ratio 2:1:100 of potassium iodide powder: iodine crystals: distilled water.

Acetone in alcohol (gram stain decolorizer)

Materials are acetone, absolute alcohol (methanol or ethanol) and distilled water. Acetone in alcohol decolorizer can be made to whatever volume by mixing materials in ratio 20:19:1 of acetone: alcohol: distilled water.

Basic carbol fuchsin (counter-stain dye)

Material are basic fuchsin powder, absolute alcohol (methanol or ethanol), phenol (powder or liquid) and distilled water. To make basic carbol fuchsin dye, materials are mixed in ratio 1:10:5:100 of basic fuchsin powder: absolute alcohol: phenol: distilled water.

Hydrochloric acid (3%) decolorizer

To make 1 liter (1000 ml), measure 30 ml of concentrated hydrochloric acid and add into 970 ml of 95% ethyl alcohol. This reagent (decolorizer) is ready to use, no further preparation is required.

Sulphuric acid (20%) decolorizer

To make 1 liter (1000 ml) of 20% sulphuric acid decolorizer, measure 200ml of concentrated sulphuric acid, add into 800 ml of distilled water. Note; acid is added into water and not vice versa.

Methylene blue (counter-stain)

Weigh 1g of methylene blue powder and add into 1000 ml of distilled water to make 1 liter (1000 ml). This solution is ready to use.

Turbidity standard solution (0.5 McFarland equivalent turbidity standard solution)

For antimicrobial susceptibility testing, inocula should be made equivalent to turbidity standard solution. Preparation of turbidity standard solution, (1) Solution 1; add 1 ml of concentrated sulphuric acid into 99 ml of distilled water. (2) Solution 2; dissolve 0.5g dehydrate barium chloride into 50 ml of distilled water. Mix 0.6 ml of solution 1 with 99.4 ml of solution 2. Dispense into small tubes of the same type of those to be used for making inocula.

Remember: All staining reagent made as explained above are stock solutions and they should be kept in amber bottles to prevent them from direct sunlight which further their deterioration. Upon their use on bench for daily procedures they should be diluted to whatever concentrations desired and they should be filtered before use to increase their quality of performance. There are commercial ready-made staining kits available, they can also be used.

Preparations of culture media
Lowenstein Jensen (LJ) medium

LJ medium is a selective medium for isolation of *Mycobacterium tuberculosis* complex (MTBC) from clinical specimens (mostly sputum) [10, 11]. MTBC requires protein enriched medium for their rapid and facilitated growth [11]. LJ medium was discovered by Lowenstein who used congo red and malachite green dyes to inhibit unwanted bacteria such as the normal flora of the upper respiratory tract system and oral cavity [10, 11]. Jensen, modified the formula to glycerated egg-based medium and by the removal of congo red while increasing the concentration of malachite green [10, 11]. Later on, Gruft modified the formula by addition of antibiotics (penicillin and nalidixic acid) and ribonucleic acid (RNA) to increase its selectivity [10, 11].

Composition of LJ medium

The key composition of LJ medium for in-house (laboratory) made includes: homogenized eggs (hen's eggs of not more than seven days old), malachite green dye (2.0 g is completely dissolved in 100 ml of distilled water), mineral salts (potassium dihydrogen phosphate anhydrous 2.4 g, magnesium sulphate anhydrous 0.24 g, magnesium citrate 0.6 g and asparagine 3.6 g which are dissolved in 600 ml of distilled water) and glycerol (favors growth of *M. tuberculosis*) or pyruvate (favors growth of *M. bovis*) [10, 11].

Cleaning and disinfecting of eggs for LJ medium.

- Eggs are soaked in soap solution for 30 minutes.
- Followed by thorough scrubbing using hand brush.
- Eggs are rinsed thoroughly in running water.
- Then, they are soaked in 70% ethanol for 15 minutes to disinfect them.
- Crack the eggs with the edge of the beaker into a sterile flask
- Using sterile (disinfected) blender, homogenize (blend) them for 30 seconds to one minute.

Preparation of complete LJ medium

- Aseptically, 600 ml of mineral salt solution, 20 ml of malachite green, 1000 ml of homogenized eggs and 12 ml of glycerol (reagent grade) are mixed together in a sterile flask.
- The medium is dispensed into universal bottles (6-8 ml) or culture bottles (14-28 ml).
- Tightly close the caps of bottles and place the bottles in slanted position on pre-heated (85℃) inspissator for 50 minutes.
- Heating on inspissator aims for solidification of medium and not for sterilization (medium was prepared under sterility conditions).

Note: too high temperature and prolonged time of stand on inspissator deteriorate the quality of egg medium.

Sterility check of LJ medium

- The whole batch of LJ media prepared should be incubated at 35°C-37°C for 24 hours to inspect for bacterial sterility.
- After 24 hours only 5% of the media randomly selected should be left for another incubation of 14 days to check for fungal sterility.

Note: contamination rate should not exceed 10%.

Screw capped bottles are used for preparation of LJ media to prevents contamination from environmental bacteria, drying out of culture media and spreading of infectious aerosols from positive cultures.

Preparation of other culture media

The instructions for preparation of other culture media such as 5% sheep blood agar, MacConkey agar or Muller Hinton agar are provided by manufacturers on their packaging tins. Therefore, preparation of these media should strictly follow manufacturer's instructions however minor modification may be made according.

Pouring of culture medium into petri dishes

For growth and isolation of bacteria on culture, the depth of medium real matters, there is an average amount of medium to be poured into petri dishes; the amount is measured into milliliter in depth after pouring of medium into petri dishes. Normally, it is not about the actual volume to be poured into petri dishes, but it is about the final depth of the poured medium into petri dishes. Because, there are different types of petri dishes with different size or volume capacities, the recommended final depth after pouring of culture medium is 4mm to 5mm. This depth will provide enough nutrients for bacterial growth while leaving enough space for bacterial colonies' not to touch the inner surface of petri dish's lid/cover. Too thin depth provides insufficient nutrient therefore limiting bacteria from growing to their actual morphology and size.

There are two major types of petri dishes, plastic (disposable) petri dishes and glass (reusable) petri dishes (Figure 3). Plastic petri dishes are cheap comparing to glass petri dishes, however in resources limited laboratories, glass petri dishes are recommended because of re-usability and once they are purchased there is no expire date unless broken.

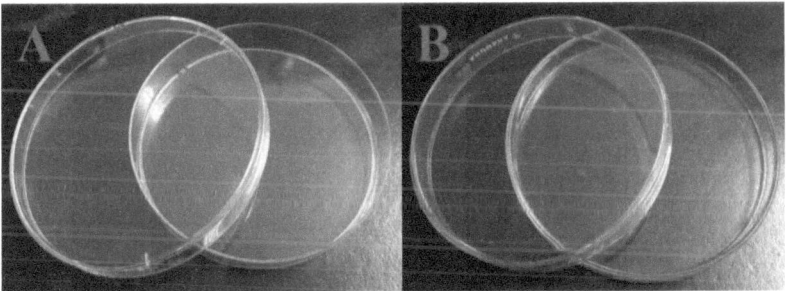

Figure 3; Petri dishes (A). Plastic (disposable) petri dish. (B). Glass (reusable) petri dish.

Laboratory quality control and assurance
Introduction

Preliminary and final reports submitted to clinicians/physicians aim to guide antimicrobial therapy for reliable management and recovery outcome of the patients. About 75% of patient management and outcome is affected by laboratory diagnosis. Proper diagnosis ensures good prognosis. Therefore, laboratory results/reports, especially culture and susceptibility should be valid (accurate and precise), hence quality must be observed throughout the first to the final procedure.

Quality control

Laboratory quality is defined as reliability and timeliness of a procedure in the laboratory. To achieve acceptable reliability, a procedure should have highest precise and accuracy. Precise is a reproducibility of a procedure's output (result) while accuracy is a closeness of a procedure's output (results) towards actual value. However, not all procedures achieve a 100% precision and 100% accuracy due to random and systematic errors, but they should be within acceptable standards, 100±1%. To ensure reliability of laboratory results, each step of a procedure, quality control should be monitored.

In Clinical Bacteriology laboratory, reagents preparation such as Gram-stain, culture media, biochemical identification media and antibiotic discs for susceptibility testing should be routinely monitored for quality.

Quality control of Gram-stain reagents/kit

Upon preparation of new batch of Gram-stain reagents or receipt of new reagents kit, quality control of these reagents is mandatory to ensure reliability. Smears of fresh culture (~24 hours) of known control organisms (*S. aureus* ATCC and *E. coli* ATCC) should be prepared on clean and greasy free microscope slides. Smeared slides are then stained adhering with local standard operating procedures for routine Gram-staining. No special attention is required because the aim is to assess reliability of; first, overall procedure and second, performance of reagents. Whenever, restraint is observed, appropriate troubleshooting of the procedural time or reagents' concentration should be addressed immediately. It is also recommended that, Gram-stain reagents/kit should be performed on weekly basis.

Quality control of culture media

Culture media are quality controlled for sterility and performance. *Sterility quality control* ensures that preparation procedures were done under sterility conditions and the prepared batch is sterile. One or two culture plate representatives, depending on the amount prepared, are randomly selected and incubated at 37 degree Celsius for 24 hours. Growth of less than two bacterial colonies per culture plate is acceptable. Growth of equal or greater than three colonies is not acceptable, the whole batch is discarded and another new batch is prepared. *Performance quality control* ensures that, expected results on culture plates are achieved. For example, hemolysis characteristics (gamma, alpha and beta) on sheep blood agar plates and lactose fermentation characteristics on MacConkey agar plates.

Quality control of conventional biochemical identification tests

Catalase, coagulase, novobiocin, bile Aesculin, bacitracin and optochin are used for differentiation and identification of Gram-positive species of Staphylococcus from/and Streptococcus respectively. Oxidase test strips, and Triple Sugar Iron (TSI), Sulfur-Indole-Motility (SIM), Simmons citrate and urease agars (tests) are used for differentiation and identifications of Gram-negative bacteria mainly of the family *Enterobacteriaceae*. Know control organisms obtained from American Type Culture Collection (ATCC), however, sub-culture of ATCC control organisms from a friend's lab or molecular typed, are recommended for controlling of biochemical identification tests. Briefly, after preparation of new batch of Gram-negative bacteria biochemical identification tests, a flesh grown *E. coli* ATCC is inoculated into prepared tests and then incubated at 37^0C for 18-24 hours or over-night. On the next day, an interpretation of these biochemical identification tests is done, expecting to get *E. coli* identified.

Quality control of antibiotic discs for susceptibility testing

Antibiotic discs for susceptibility testing may deteriorate on exposure to high temperature; most of the time this is happening during transportations to remote areas where thawing of ice-packs is inevitable due to time factor. Therefore, upon receipt of new antibiotic discs for susceptibility testing, they should be quality checked for performance. Briefly, inoculum of control organisms (*S. aureus* ATCC 25923 or *E. coli* ATCC 25922) should be prepared form flesh grown culture (about 24 hours) equivalent to 0.5MacFarland turbidity standard solution and then swabbed on entire Muller Hinton agar (MHA) plate. Antibiotic discs to be quality checked are then seeded and plate(s) is incubated at 37^{0}C for 18-24 hours. An interpretation of zones of inhibitions is done on the next day as guided by Clinical and Laboratory Standard Institute (CLSI) guideline for control organisms. Any antibiotic disc which will not pass this control test should be omitted from routine use for patients' bacteria susceptibility testing because they will mislead patients' treatment.

Conventional bacteriological culture
Introduction

In laboratories with limited resources, conventional clinical bacteriology can be carried out for routinely isolation of anaerobic pathogens from clinical specimens. Clinical specimens like blood, urine, stool, pus and sputum can be inoculated onto appropriate culture media for diagnosis of blood stream infection, urinary tract infection, gastroenteritis, skin and soft tissue infections and lower respiratory tract infection respectively. Significant bacteria isolated from these specimens should undergo further procedures including conventional (in-house) biochemical identifications testing and antibiotic susceptibility testing to guide rational therapy.

Urine culture

Urine is sterile specimen from urinary tract system. It is used for diagnosis of urinary tract infections (UTIs) [12]. UTI is categorized into; pyelonephritis, infection of the kidneys and cystis, infection of the urinary bladder [13, 14]. The most common pathogens causing UTI are; gram negative bacteria, *Escherichia coli*, *Klebsiella pneumoniae*, *Klebsiella oxytoca*, *Proteus vurgalis*, *Proteus mirabillis* and *Pseudomonas aeruginosa* [15, 16]. Gram positive bacteria are, *Staphylococcus aureus*, *Staphylococcus saprophyticus*, *Enterococcus faecalis* and *Streptococcus pyogenes* [15, 16]. Fungal species commonly associated with UTI is *Candida albicans* [15, 16]. Growth of Coagulase Negative *Staphylococci* (CoNS), *Viridans streptococci*, *Corynebacterium* spp., and *Lactobacillus* spp is considered as contamination, however can be determined as significant regarding colony count and clinical presentations of specific individual patient [17]. Growth of bacteria from urine culture is termed as bacteriuria and growth of fungi from urine culture is termed as fungiuria.

The best type of urine specimen for culture and sensitivity is mid-stream catch urine [18]. Mid-stream catch urine is collected after cleaning of external genitalia (in women) with clean running water, patient void to the toilet but holding the mid-stream which he/she urinate into sterile urine container and then finish voiding to the toilet [19]. The first stream aims to clean urethra and reduce the chance of contaminating specimen with some normal flora of the skin [19]. Another types of urine specimens are, supra-pubic urine specimen and catheterized urine specimen [20]. Supra-pubic urine specimen is collected directly from patient's urinary bladder through supra-pubic region by aspiration using sterile needle and syringe after locating of

119

bladder by palpation and aid of ultra-sound. This type of urine specimen is collected from patients who are unable of self-voiding and whose urethra is blocked and the insertion of catheter tube is not possible. Supra-pubic urine specimen should be collected by skilled clinicians. Catheterized urine specimen is collected from patients with indwelling catheters. Catheter tube is disinfected and clamped to trap the flow stream of urine from urinary bladder and then needle and syringe is used to aspirate the trapped urine within catheter tube. Urine from catheter bag is not recommended as it can have been stayed for a long time and it is known that urine is nutritious like culture medium, it enhance rapid multiplication of microorganisms that giving false quantity on laboratory culture [21].

Urine should be processed within two hours after collection to avoid false positive results as long staying urine specimen at room temperature acts as culture medium to facilitate multiplication of bacteria present in the specimens [21]. If delay in urine processing is inevitable, refrigeration should be considered at 2 to 8 degree Celsius [22].

Processing of urine for culture

Macroscopic examination; considering color (e.g colorless, yellowish, amber) and consistency or turbidity of urine specimen (e.g clear or turbid) [23].

Microscopic examination; wet preparation and smear for gram stain. In wet preparation, the presence of inflammatory cells, while blood cells is considered and in gram stain the presence of microorganisms is considered [23, 24].

Urine chemistry (Urine dip stick); by using dip stick, presence of leucocytes, nitrites and urine ph are measured [25]. Leucocytes are inflammatory cells; their presence in urine signifies the presence of infection. Nitrite is converted from nitrate by bacteria in the family Enterobacteriaceae; presence of nitrite signifies presence of bacteria in urine specimen. Most often, bacterial infection of the urinary tract is favored by alkalinity condition of the urine [26].

Inoculation of urine samples on culture media

Appropriate selection of culture media for urine is very essential. In resources limited settings, C.L.E.D (cysteine lactose electrolyte deficient) culture medium is enough [27]. It is general, allows growth of gram negative and positive bacteria and differential, it differentiate between lactose fermenters and none lactose fermenters. C.L.E.D medium is recommended as it inhibits the swarming characteristics of *Proteus* spp as it does on sheep blood agar (SBA). But, sheep blood agar (SBA) for growth of gram positive and gram negative bacteria and MacConkey agar (MCA) for growth of gram negative bacteria and also a differential medium for lactose fermentation characteristic can be used. Whenever, fungal infection is suspected, Sabraud dextrose agar (SDA) is recommended. Culture plates should be aerobically incubated at 37^{0}C for 24-48 hours.

Urine culture is done quantitatively by using calibrated wire loops of 10µl in diameter (Figure 1). First, streaks straight line from top to bottom of culture plate when held vertically and then streaking perpendicular lines across the first straight streaking line. These streaking patterns allow evenly distribution of bacteria colonies of culture plate enhancing counting of colony forming units. Interpretation of culture results on culture media include the quantity of bacteria forming colonies grown on specific culture medium [17]. Growth equal to or greater than ten power five colonies forming unit per one milliliter of urine ($\geq 10^5$ CFU/ml) is considered significant [17]. Thereafter, biochemical identification of isolated bacteria to species level and antibiotic susceptibility testing follows. However, growth of greater than or equal to ten power three colonies forming unit per one milliliter of urine ($\geq 10^3$ CFU/ml) is considered significant whenever the patients is presenting with clinical symptoms [17]. Growth of less than ten power three colonies forming unit per one milliliter of urine ($^< 10^3$ CFU/ml) is considered not significant.

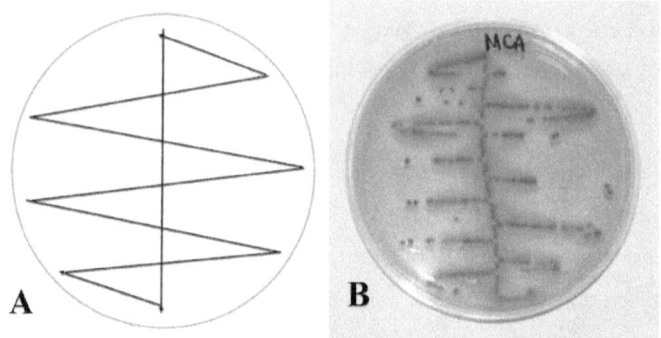

Figure 3; Urine culture for quantification (A). Showing culture patterns for urine specimen. (B). Showing lactose fermenting colonies (pinkish colonies) on MCA.

Calculation of colonies forming unit (CFU)

Count exact number of colonies grown on culture medium using 10µl wire loop, and then convert that number into 1ml of urine specimen to get X CFU/ml.

Example; 150 colonies has grown on C.L.E.D

10 µl of urine = 150 colonies

1 ml of urine = x colonies

But, 1 ml of urine = 1000 µl of urine

10x µl = 150 colonies x 1000 µl

X = (150 colonies x 1000 µl) ÷ 10 µl

X = 15000 colonies = 1.5×10^4 CFU/ml

10^4 CFU/ml

After quantifying exact number of bacteria grown on culture plate, biochemical identification testing is done (discussed under Chapter three) for significant growth and for pathogenic bacteria, antibiotic susceptibility testing is done (discussed under Chapter four) to guide clinicians' management of the patients.

Bench aid for urine culture

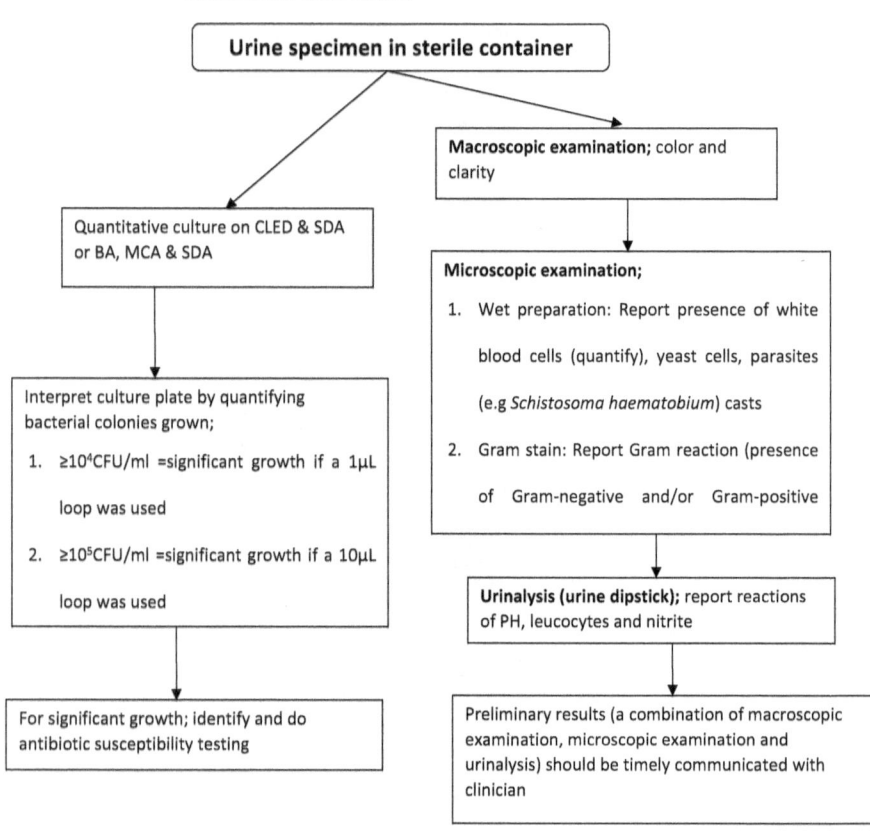

Urine specimen in sterile container

Macroscopic examination; color and clarity

Quantitative culture on CLED & SDA or BA, MCA & SDA

Microscopic examination;

1. Wet preparation: Report presence of white blood cells (quantify), yeast cells, parasites (e.g *Schistosoma haematobium*) casts

2. Gram stain: Report Gram reaction (presence of Gram-negative and/or Gram-positive

Interpret culture plate by quantifying bacterial colonies grown;

1. $\geq 10^4$CFU/ml =significant growth if a 1µL loop was used

2. $\geq 10^5$CFU/ml =significant growth if a 10µL loop was used

Urinalysis (urine dipstick); report reactions of PH, leucocytes and nitrite

For significant growth; identify and do antibiotic susceptibility testing

Preliminary results (a combination of macroscopic examination, microscopic examination and urinalysis) should be timely communicated with clinician

Blood culture

Blood is another sterile specimen, free from microorganisms as resident or normal flora. Blood for culture aims to isolate sepsis causative microorganism [16]. The most common pathogens are; *Escherichia coli*, *Klebsiella pneumoniae*, *Acinetobacter* spp., *Staphylococcus aureus*, *Salmonella* spp., *Pseudomonas aeruginosa* and *Proteus* spp [15, 16, 28]. Most likely contaminants are skin normal flora, Coagulase Negative Staphylococci (CoNS) and Viridans streptococci, *Micrococcus* and *Bacillus* spp [15, 28]. Blood specimen for culture and sensitivity is collected when sepsis is suspected due to presence of clinical symptoms and signs; fever, chills, comma and difficulty in breathing (esp. in neonates) [16]. Bacterial toxins is responsible for symptoms presentation [16]. Growth of bacteria in blood for asymptomatic patient is termed as bacteremia while for symptomatic patient is termed as septicemia.

Conventional blood culture system

Conventional blood culture involves the use of in-house made blood culture bottles (vials) which are conventionally incubated in a normal incubators used for incubation of other inoculated culture media. Signs of microorganisms' growth and activities are observed visibly by naked eyes on daily basis for up to seven days of incubation.

Collection of blood for culture [29-31]

- As blood is sterile specimen, so does collection of blood for culture and sensitivity should be sterile procedures. None sterile procedure may contaminate blood specimen with skin normal flora and/or ubiquitous environment bacteria.
- Procedures for collection of blood for culture and sensitivity
- Assemble all equipment and materials required for collection of blood for culture
- Introduce the procedure to be done to the patient
- Tie a tourniquet at the upper arm of the patient aiming for median cubital vein
- Wear clean sterile gloves
- Concentrically disinfect the site of vein puncture (from center to periphery with circular motion) by using bactericidal disinfectant eg. 70% alcohol, 2% tincture of iodine and 10% povidone-iodine

- Withdraw blood from the patient by using recommended needle and syringe considering age of the patient
- Make sure to disinfect top of culture bottle before inserting needle and syringe for injecting blood specimen into culture bottle
- Mix well blood and broth in blood culture bottle by 8 to 10 inversions

Remember: Volume of blood to withdraw with age; 1-2.5ml neonates, 2.5-5ml children and 5-10ml adults [16]. Recommended broth for blood for culture is tryptic soy broth (TSB) or brain heart infusion broth (BHIB). Ratio of blood to broth should be 1:10 [31, 32]. Broth functions to multiply the few microorganisms present in blood as they can be few but presenting symptoms to patients as a result of their toxins. Blood for culture and sensitivity should be collected before administration of antibiotic and it is recommended to collect two specimens for the same patient when fever is high [31-33].

Blood culture bottles are incubated at 37 degree Celsius for a follow up of seven days monitoring growth indicators; turbidity, hemolysis, production of gas and pellicles (a result of bacterial biofilm formation) on surface or bottom of the bottle (figure 4) [31]. Upon observation of growth indicator(s), blood is sub-cultured onto solid culture media. But blood should blindly sub-culture onto solid culture media day seven whenever there is no growth indicator(s).

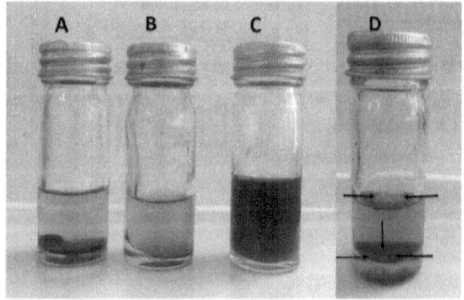

Figure 4: In-house made blood culture bottles by using Brain Heart Infusion (BHI) broth. (A); clear broth, no sign of growth, (B); turbid broth, (C); hemolysis and (D); pellicles on bottom and surface of the broth, shown by arrows

BACTEC blood culture system

Significantly, BACTEC blood culture system has higher detection rate of microorganisms with mean time of 48 hours as compared to conventional blood culture system [34].

Before using of BACTEC blood bottles (vials), they are inspected for contamination, cracks or any other sign deterioration [35]. Basically, contamination is by observing the clarity of broth inside the vial. Any vial with turbid broth is not recommended for use. After patient's preparation for vein-puncture to withdraw blood specimen, flip caps of two BACTEC vials (aerobic and anaerobic vials) are removed followed by disinfection of the top of vials by using 70% alcohol [35]. The use of iodine is not recommended. Then, vials' tops are left to air dry before inoculating blood specimen. Blood specimen is inoculated in BACTEC vials up to the fill-mark on vials. Aerobic BACTEC vial is inoculated first followed by anaerobic BCTEC vial [35]. The volume of blood specimen to be inoculated depends on patient's age and type of BACTEC vial (e.g., neonate, children or adult vial). Vials are labeled accordingly as per requisition form and then sent to Bacteriology laboratory in cool box at room temperature.

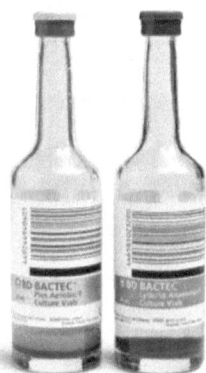

**Figure 5: BD BACTEC blood culture vials, left for aerobic and right for anaerobic culture
(Source: DUFORT ET LAVIGNE)**

In laboratory, BACTEC vials are incubated in BACTEC machine at 37℃ for a follow up of 7 days until the machine flips for detection of growth. Detection of positive growth is followed by Gram stain and sub-culture of solid culture media as per standard operating procedures of the specific laboratory.

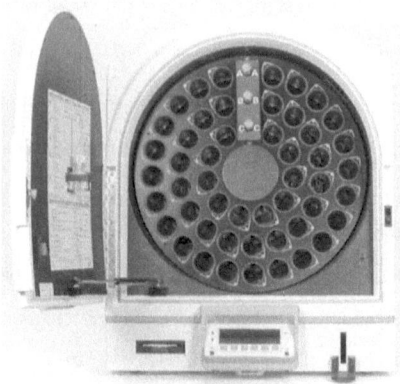

Figure 6: BD BACTEC 9050 (Source: Artisan Technology Group)

Inoculation (sub-culture) of blood samples on solid culture media

Selection of appropriate solid culture media; sheep blood agar (SBA), MacConkey agar (MCA) and Sabraud dextrose agar (SDA) when fungal infection is suspected are used for sub-culture. Streaking patterns for blood specimens is shown in figure 5. Blood culture is not done quantitatively as urine because of in vitro multiplication of microorganisms in blood specimen. Culture plates are incubated in 37 degree Celsius for 18-24 hours.

Bacterial growth on solid culture plates is interpreted by considering colonies' growth morphology and characteristics. For significant growth, biochemical identification of bacterial to species level and antibiotic susceptibility testing follows.

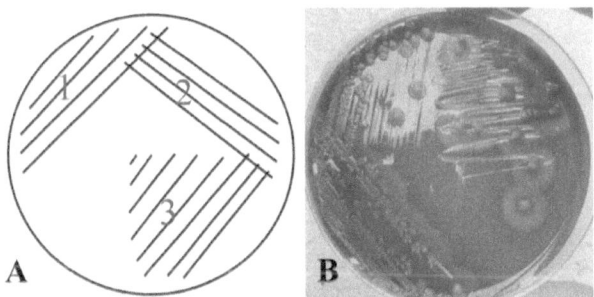

Figure 7; Blood culture patterns. (A). Showing streaking patterns on culture plate medium. (B). Sheep blood agar showing bacteria colonies with beta hemolysis.

Bench aid for blood culture

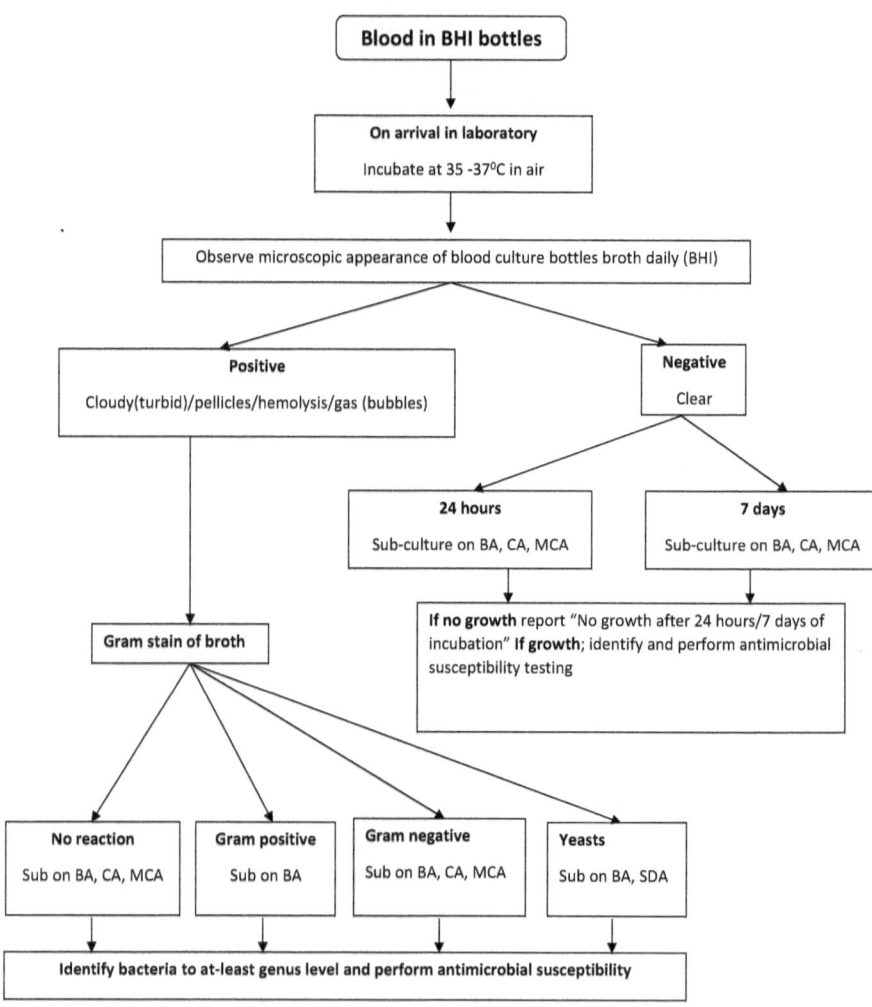

Pus culture

Pus specimen can be from surgical site infection (SSI), infected none surgical wounds and exudates [36, 37]. Accumulation of pus in wound or body cavity such as peritoneum, pericardium is known as exudate [38]. The most common pathogens are, *Pseudomonas aeruginosa, Acinetobacter* spp., *Escherichia coli, Klebsiella pneumoniae, Staphylococcus aureus, Streptococcus pyogenes* and *Mycobacterium tuberculosis*(causing extra-pulmonary tuberculosis) [38, 39]. Group D streptococcus, *Staphylococcus epidermidis* (skin normal flora) and none pathogenic *Bacillus* spp from environment and surfaces can contaminate pus specimen if improperly collected.

Collection of pus specimen can be done by using sterile cotton swab in Stuart transport medium (figure 3) if discharge is not in excess [40, 41]. For deep seated and exudates, aspiration by using needle and syringe is recommended [41].

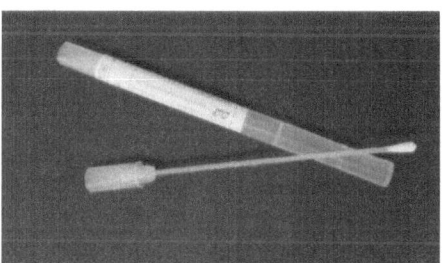

Figure 8; Swab with Stuart transport medium (Guangzhou, China)

Processing of pus specimen

Macroscopic examination; color and odour of the specimen is considered. Color can predict the most likely pathogen to be isolated, for example greenish pus is suggestive of *Pseudomonas aeruginosa* infection as these species produces greenish pigments known as pyoverdin [42]. Other types of color can be yellowish, yellow-brownish or brownish. Most often pus specimens from anaerobic pathogens has foul smell [43]. But in this book, aerobic culture only will be discussed.

Microscopic examination, gram stain and modified ZN stain [44]. Gram staining of pus specimen is done to examine the presence of bacteria as preliminary results. Modified ZN staining is done to examine the presence of Mycobacterium tuberculosis in case of extra-pulmonary tuberculosis.

Culture of pus specimen; recommended culture media are sheep blood agar (SBA), chocolate agar (CA-should be incubated micro-aerophilically) and MacConkey agar (MCA). Streaking pattern is by three quadrants and if quantification is necessary, it is done by considering growth on first, second and third streaking quadrants as +1, +2 and +3 (refer figure 2). Significant growth of bacteria is identified to species level and antibacterial susceptibility testing is done to guide rational treatment.

Bench aid for pus culture

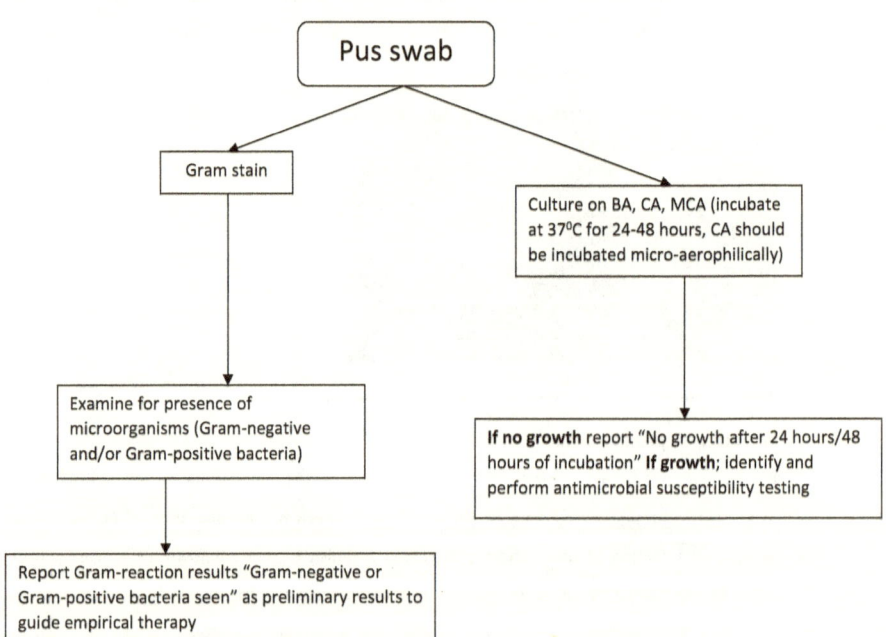

Stool culture

Stool specimen is used to diagnose infections of the gastro-intestinal tract (GIT). Routine pathogens in bacteriology laboratory are *Salmonella* spp causing typhoid fever and *Shigella* spp causing gastro-enteritis (diarrhea and bloody diarrhea) [16]. Stool specimen for culture and sensitivity should be collected in sterile container, if analysis will not delay, transport medium is not necessary however Cary Blair transport medium can be used [45]. This medium is semi-solid in nature and has less nutrients purposely, not to allow bacterial multiplication but keeping them viable till culture is done. Other transport medium which can be used with stool specimens are alkaline peptone water and Selenite F broth [46, 47]. Alkaline peptone water is used for transportation of stool specimen from cholera suspect and Selenite F is used for enrichment of *Salmonella* spp and *Shigella* spp while inhibiting GIT normal flora [46, 47].

Processing of stool specimens

Macroscopic examination; color and texture of specimen are very important. Deviation of color from normal, brownish (adult) may be due to infection however diet can contribute to stool specimen color change, for example greenish specimen after vegetables containing meal or creamy (breastfeed children). Color may be, brownish, yellowish, and blackish. Texture includes; watery or loose, semi-solid or semi-formed and solid or formed stool specimen. Stool may contain mucus or blood, should be reported as well [9].

Microscopic examination; gram staining and modified ZN staining may be employed [7]. Stool specimen contain numbers of GIT normal flora but some pathogens have peculiar morphology specifically identify them under microscope with gram stain, even single diluted (1-3%) carbol fuchsin can work out. For example, gram negative and comma shaped rods are *Vibrio* spp, gram negative "C" or "S" shaped rods are *Campylobacter* spp and gram positive rods with terminal spores "drum stick" are *Clostridium difficile* causative agent of pseudo membranous colitis (Figure 7 & 8). However sensitivity and specificity of direct gram stain in detection of gastroenteritis causing pathogens varies from 60% to 90% depending endemicity and experience of laboratory personnel, but still can be used to provide preliminary results whenever treatment of the patient cannot be delayed and to guide culture results. For identification of *Cryptosporidium parvum* causing diarrhea and wasting among immunocompromised patients with HIV/AIDS positive, *Isospora belli* and *Cyclospora* spp oocysts, modified ZN stain is used [7].

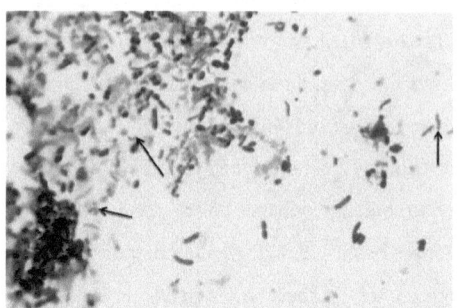

Figure 9; *Campylobacter* **spp, "C" and "S" shaped gram negative rods shown by black arrows (image source; Mushi FM** *et al,.* **2014)**

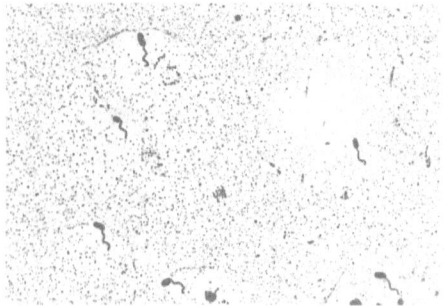

Figure 10; Comma shaped gram negative bacteria of *Vibrio* **spp (image source; Lumen, Boundless Microbiology, Bacterial diseases of the digestive system)**

Inoculation of stool samples on culture media

Stool culture is done on Salmonella Shigella agar (SSA), thiosulfate-citrate-bile salt-sucrose agar (TCBS), or modified charcoal-cefoperazone-deoxycholate ager (Modified-CCDA) depending on interest of diagnosis.

For the isolation of *Salmonella* spp and *Shigella* spp causing typhoid fever and dysentery respectively, SSA is used [48]. Before culture is done on SSA it should be inoculated in Selenite F broth for at least six hours and then sub-cultured onto SSA [48]. Colonies of *Salmonella* spp on SSA have black centers while *Shigella* spp give colorless colonies (Figure 9). These characteristics on SSA they should not be used as confirmatory identification for *Salmonella* spp and *Shigella* as long as *Proteus* spp if managed to grow on SSA they also give blackish colonies [49]. Biochemical identification tests to identify bacteria to species level are mandatory. After identification of pathogen causing infection of the GIT, antibiotic susceptibility testing is done.

CHROMagar for isolation of *Salmonella* and *Shigella* spp can also be used if available. The advantage of CHROMagar over SSA is high sensitivity and there is no need of using biochemical identification tests as CHROMagar identifies *Salmonella* and *Shigella* isolates to their species level chromatographically hence cost effective [50].

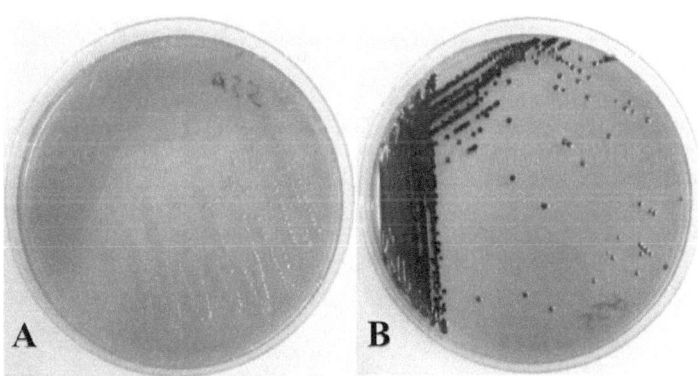

Figure 11; Salmonella Shigella agar (SSA) (A); none pigmenting colonies on SSA most likely *Shigella* spp., (B). Sulphur pigmenting colonies, blackish at the center most likely *Salmonella* spp.

For the isolation of *Vibrio cholera* from presumptive patient with cholera, TCBS is used which is selectively isolate *V. cholera* and differentiate it from other *Vibrio* species viz. *V. parahemolyticus* by yellowish coloration of *V. cholera* colonies [51]. Fermentation of sucrose sugar in TCBS by *V. cholera* result in growth of yellowish colonies, therefore, interpretation of culture plates should be done immediately because as plates stay on room temperature yellow colonies reverts to green color [51]. Vomitus, food remnant, watery diarrhea and/or environmental specimen such as water in sterile specimen container should be enriched in alkaline-peptone water to facilitate rapid multiplication of *V. cholera* while inhibiting other enteric bacteria which may interfere isolation of *V. cholera*. Bile salts and high pH of TCBS makes it selective [52]. Bile salts inhibit growth of Gram-positive bacteria while high pH (8.5-9.5) inhibits growth of other enteric bacteria [52]. TCBS plates should be incubated aerobically at 37°C for 24-48 hours.

Isolation of *Campylobacter* species from presumptive diarrheagenic patients is done on Modified-CCDA [53]. This culture medium contains cefoperazone which makes it selective and amphotericin B which inhibit growth of yeast and fungi. *Campylobacter coli*, *Campylobacter jejuni* and *Campylobacter laridis* can be isolated using Modified-CCDA. Colonies of *Campylobacter* species appear grey in color, moist and flat spreading with or without metallic sheen however colonies of *C. coli* are slightly raised. *Campylobacter* species are microaerophilic, therefore culture plates should be incubated in candle jar at 37°C for 48 hours [53].

Cerebral spinal fluid (CSF) culture
CSF is a core specimen in diagnosis of meninges infections (meningitis) [54]. The most common bacteria causing meningitis are *Escherichia coli*, *Listeria monocytogens* and *Streptococcus agalactiae* (in neonates) and *Neisseria meningitidis*, *Streptococcus pneumoniae*, *Haemophilus influenza* type b, *Listeria monocytogens*, *Treponema pallidum* and *Mycobacterium tuberculosis* (other age groups) [15, 54]. CSF should be processed urgently because meningitis is a critical life threatening infection and cellular materials in CSF specimen degenerate very rapid which can result to false negative laboratory results [16]. Do not refrigerate or freeze CSF specimen [55].

Processing of CSF specimen
Macroscopic examination, color and turbidity of CSF specimen are considered. A normal CSF is clear and colorless [44]. Any deviation of the color indicates inflammation, except blood containing CSF which may indicate hemorrhage during specimen collection or at certain part of the meninges. Turbid CSF also indicates the presence of inflammation due to infection of the meninges [16, 44].

Microscopic examination, direct microscopy, India ink stain, gram stain and ZN stain are performed [56-58]. Direct microscopy, a drop of CSF specimen is examined under microscope for the presence of blood cells, white blood cells (WBC) and red blood cells (RBC) are aimed. India ink aims to detect the presence of encapsulated yeast cells of *Cryptococcus neoformans*, a common pathogen among immunocompromised (eg. HIV/AIDS) patients [59, 60]. Gram stain aims to detect the presence of either gram negative bacteria or gram positive bacteria causing meningitis. ZN stain is aimed for the detection of *Mycobacterium tuberculosis* causing extra-pulmonary tuberculosis [56].

CSF chemistry, glucose and protein are examined. Glucose is reduced if the etiological agent is bacteria because bacteria utilize sugars but normal for viral meningitis [16, 44]. Protein is elevated in all kind of infections, bacterial meningitis and viral meningitis [16, 44].

Culture of CSF specimen

CSF culture should be done on sheep blood agar (SBA), chocolate agar (CA) and MacConkey agar (MCA) aiming gram positive bacteria, fastidious bacteria and gram negative bacteria causing bacterial meningitis respectively. All culture media are incubated at 35-37 degree Celsius however; SBA and CA should be incubated in candle jar with a burning candle in it to enrich the environment with carbon dioxide to favor growth of micro-aerophilic bacteria eg. *Streptococcus agalactiae* and *Neisseria meningitidis*. Significant growth of bacteria should be identified to species level followed by antimicrobial susceptibility testing for patient's rational therapy. If possible, culture of CSF on Lowenstein Jensen (LJ) medium should be performed for detection of tuberculous meningitis (TBM) as culture remain the gold standard technique [56].

Blood culture system for body fluid specimens

In recent years, the use of blood culture system for other sterile body fluids such as CSF, pleural effusion, ascites, or joint fluid is increasing and acceptable [61, 62]. This system has been shown to improve the overall recovery of bacteria because it is more sensitive than conventional culture methods [61, 62]. The conventional culture methods of body fluid uses a solid media for culture, and sometime before inoculating bacteria on solid culture media, various procedures such as filtration and centrifugation are required to concentrate the organism [61]. Additionally, it is just a small volume of sample is inoculated on solid culture media carrying very few microorganisms if any, therefore lowering its sensitivity in isolating of the bacteria [61]. Blood culture bottles contain nutritious broth which facilitates growth and multiplication of the very few bacteria in body fluid [61]. Moreover, broth fluid in blood culture bottles neutralizes antibiotics which might inhibit the recovery of bacteria if they were to be inoculated directly on solid culture media [61].

Bench aid for CSF processing

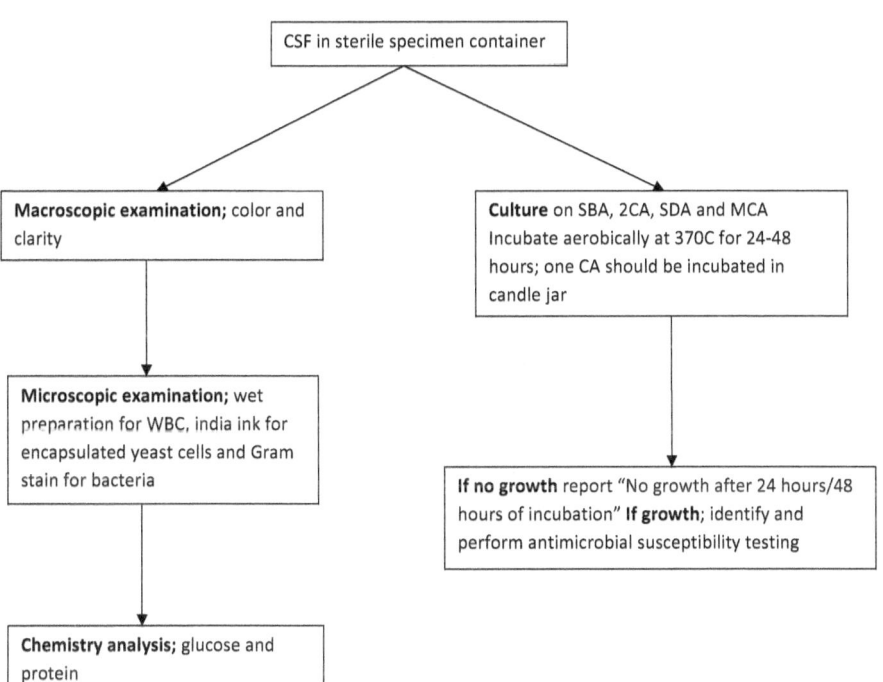

CSF in sterile specimen container

Macroscopic examination; color and clarity

Culture on SBA, 2CA, SDA and MCA Incubate aerobically at 370C for 24-48 hours; one CA should be incubated in candle jar

Microscopic examination; wet preparation for WBC, india ink for encapsulated yeast cells and Gram stain for bacteria

If no growth report "No growth after 24 hours/48 hours of incubation" **If growth**; identify and perform antimicrobial susceptibility testing

Chemistry analysis; glucose and protein

Respiratory tract specimens' culture

Respiratory tract is marked from nostrils to alveolar sacs through respiratory tubes and it is divided into two systems, upper respiratory and lower respiratory tracts bounded at larynx [63, 64]. The most common bacterial infection of upper respiratory tract system is otitis media, sinusitis and tonsillitis [63, 64]. Tonsillitis caused by *Streptococcus pyogenes* [63]will be discussed under this chapter. Bacterial infections of the lower respiratory tract systems are categorized into tuberculous and none-tuberculous infections. Tuberculous infection is known as pulmonary tuberculosis and is caused by *Mycobacterium tuberculosis* [65, 66]. The most frequently none-tuberculous infections is pneumoniae and the most common implicating etiologies are *Streptococcus pneumoniae*, *Klebsiella pneumoniae*, *Pseudomonas aeruginosa*, *Proteus* spp., *Mycoplasma pneumoniae*, *Escherichia coli* and *Haemophilus influenza* type b [67, 68]. Bacteriological investigation of tonsillitis, pneumoniae and tuberculosis will be discussed in detail under this part. Specimen for tonsillitis is swab in Stuart transport medium while for lower respiratory tract infections is sputum. The upper respiratory tract system is none sterile, containing numbers of normal flora bacteria, *Viridans streptococci*, *Staphylococcus aureus*, *Staphylococcus epidermidis*, *Bacillus* spp, *Corynebacterium* spp., *Micrococcus* spp., and *Stomatococcus* spp [69]. The lower respiratory tract system is sterile, but when sputum specimens are passing through upper respiratory tract system during collection, it is become contaminated with upper respiratory tract system's normal flora.

Processing of sputum specimen

Upper respiratory tract specimen, sterile bacteriological swab is used to collect specimen from inflamed tonsils. Swab is transported in Stuart transport medium to the laboratory. In bacteriology laboratory, culture is done on sheep blood agar (SBA) and MacConkey agar (MCA) followed by gram staining smear for examining the presence of Polymorph nuclear (PMN) cells.

Sputum is a common specimen for diagnosis of lower respiratory tract infections, tuberculous and none-tuberculous. Sputum processing is passing through, macroscopic examination, microscopic examination and culture.

Macroscopic examination, sputum can be muco-salivary (mucus containing saliva), mucoid (pure mucus), muco-purulent (mucus containing pus) and purulent (pure pus) [15]. Sputum specimen can also contain blood or it can be rust-like appearance or greenish colored [70].

Rust-like appearance signifies pneumococcal pneumoniae due to *Streptococcus pneumoniae* [71, 72]. Greenish coloration of sputum is due to massive destruction of neutrophil cells and the release of myeloperoxidase enzymes within these cells [73]. Greenish sputum signifies one among the following, cystic fibrosis, bronchiectasis or chronic pneumoniae [74]. Common sputum color for tuberculous infection may be red, brown or black [74].

Microscopic examination: two smears for gram staining and ZN staining. Gram stain is done for examination of Polymorph nuclear (PMN) cells and ZN stain is done for microscopic diagnosis of acid fast bacilli causing tuberculosis infection.

Culture of sputum specimen

Culture for pneumonia infection is done on sheep blood agar (SBA), chocolate agar (CA) and MacConkey agar (MCA). Incubation of SBA is done in candle jar with a burning candle and optochin disc can directly be incorporated during primary culture to facilitate growth and pre-identification of *S. pneumoniae*. CA is used for the isolation of fastidious bacteria, *Haemophilus influenza* type b and MCA is used for the isolation of gram negative bacteria. Culture for tuberculous infection for the isolation of *Mycobacterium tuberculosis* is done on Lowenstein Jensen (LJ) medium, a gold standard technique [56].

Significant growth of bacteria on SBA, CA or MCA is biochemically identified (discussed under Chapter Three) to species level and antimicrobial susceptibility testing (discussed under Chapter Four) is also done to guide patient's rational therapy.

Bench aid for processing of sputum specimens

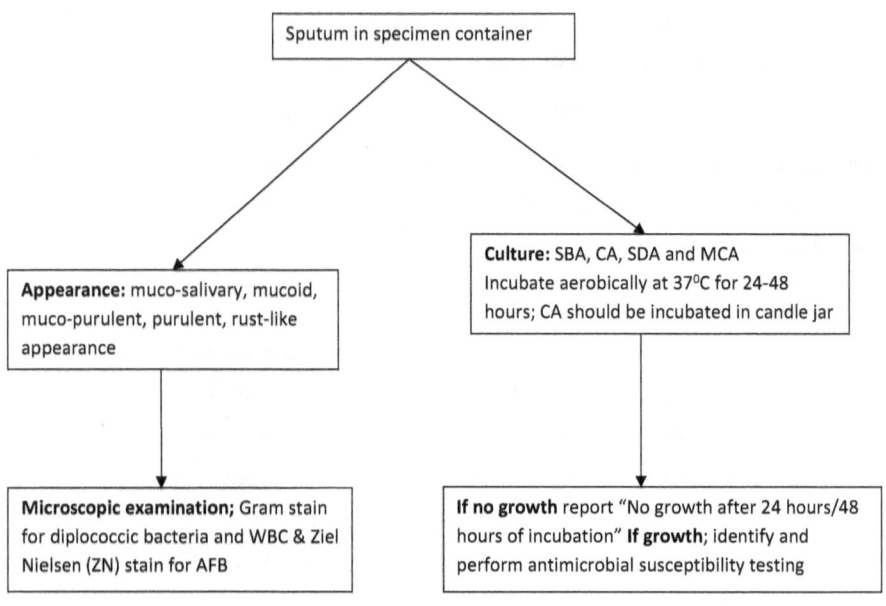

Sputum in specimen container

Appearance: muco-salivary, mucoid, muco-purulent, purulent, rust-like appearance

Culture: SBA, CA, SDA and MCA
Incubate aerobically at 37⁰C for 24-48 hours; CA should be incubated in candle jar

Microscopic examination; Gram stain for diplococcic bacteria and WBC & Ziel Nielsen (ZN) stain for AFB

If no growth report "No growth after 24 hours/48 hours of incubation" **If growth**; identify and perform antimicrobial susceptibility testing

Culture of bone and tissue biopsies

Sometime culture of drainage or discharge from infected deep seated tissues or bones (in the case of osteomyelitis) is ambiguous because in most cases, only superficial skin contaminating bacteria are isolated. Therefore, to determine true pathogens responsible for such particular infections, culture of tissue or bone biopsy is necessary [75, 76].

It is recommended two tissue or bone biopsy samples be obtained from each patient (or infection in case of multiple infections) during standard or surgical procedures as per accepted guidelines. One sample is placed in standard transport medium (e.g., Port-a-germ; Biomérieux) and another is placed in broth medium (e.g., brain heart infusion, thioglycolate broth, nutrient broth, rosenow broth or tryptic soy broth), and then, immediately transported to the laboratory for bacteriological processing [77, 78].

In the laboratory, sample in transport medium is aseptically crushed and inoculated onto appropriate culture media including two plates of 5% sheep blood agar media of which one will be incubated aerobically and the other will be incubated anaerobically at 37°C for 24-72 hours [77, 78]. Sample in broth medium is incubated in ambient air at 37°C for overnight and then it should be sub-cultured (after gently mixing) onto appropriate culture media with one 5% sheep blood agar plate being incubated anaerobically [77, 78]. Broth tubes containing tissue or bone biopsy are incubated for 7 days with daily inspection of any sign of growth including turbidity, or presences of gas bubbles or pellicles [77].

Isolated pathogen is identified to species level and then antibiotics susceptibility testing is performed as per standard operating procedures of specific laboratory.

Conventional biochemical identification of bacteria
Introduction

A combination set of conventional biochemical tests' results is used for identification of bacteria to species level or at-least to genus level. However, selection of biochemical identification tests should be guided by Gram-stain reaction of the specific bacteria. At a minimum; triple sugar iron agar, sulfur-indole-motility agar, simmons citrate agar, urease agar and oxidase strips can be used for identification of Gram-negative bacteria in the family Enterobacteriaceae while catalase (hydrogen peroxide reagent), coagulase (rabbit plasma), novobiocin disc, bacitracin disc, optochin disc and bile Aesculin can be used to identify Gram-positive bacteria specifically *Staphylococcus*, *Streptococcus* and *Enterococcus* species.

Selection of biochemical identification tests rely on gram reaction (gram stain results) of the specific bacteria grown on culture medium due to specificity with gram reaction of some biochemical identification tests. For example triple sugar iron (TSI) agar is only used for identification of gram negative bacteria.

Identification of gram positive bacteria
Identification of common *Staphylococcus* spp pathogens

Catalase test

This test is used to differentiate the bacteria that produce the enzymes catalase, such as *Staphylococcus* spp from non-catalase producing bacteria such as *Streptococcus* spp. Under microscope gram stained, *Staphylococcus* spp are gram positive cocci in clusters while *Streptococcus* spp are gram positive cocci in chains [15, 79].

Principle of catalase test

Catalase acts as catalyst in the breakdown of hydrogen peroxide to oxygen and water.

Procedure for catalase test

- Pour 1 ml of hydrogen peroxidase (H_2O_2) into test tube or a drop of H_2O_2 on a clean glass slide
- Using sterile stick, remove a good growth of test organism then immerse into H2O2 solution in test tube

- Look for immediate bubbling

Results reporting

- Bubbles- catalase positive
- No bubbles- catalase negative

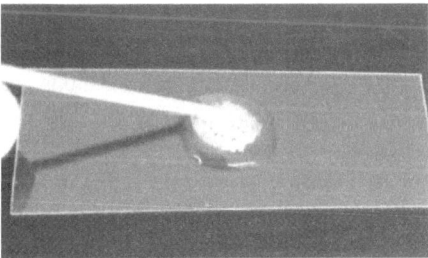

Figure 12; A positive catalase test, formation of bubbles by catalase positive bacteria on hydrogen peroxide.

Coagulase test

This test is used to differentiate *Staphylococcus aureus* form other spp of *Staphylococcus* as *Staphylococcus aureus* produce coagulase enzymes but other *Staphylococcus* spp does not [15, 79].

Principle of coagulase test

Coagulase causes plasma to clot by converting fibrinogen into fibrin

Procedures for coagulase test

- Take 3 test tubes and label them as T (test organism), P (positive control) an N (negative control)
- Pipette 0.2 ml of plasma into each test tube
- Suspend 3 to 5 colonies of test organism into test tube T, suspend 3 to 5 colonies of S aureus ATCC 25923 into test tube P and add 0.8 ml of sterile normal saline to the tube N
- Gently mix the mixture in three tubes and incubate at 35-37°C for 1 hour
- Examine for clotting formation, if after 1 hour tube T is negative then leave the tubes overnight

Results reporting for coagulase test

Clot formed- coagulase positive

No clotting- coagulase negative

Novobiocin disc test

This disc is used to identify *Staphylococcus saprophyticus* from *Staphylococcus epidermidis*. *S. saprophyticus* is resistant while *S. epidermidis* is sensitive to Novobiocin disc [15, 79].

Identification of common *Streptococcus* spp pathogens

Streptococcus spp are Lancefield classified, groups A, B, and D are of health important. Identification of common pathogens of *Streptococcus* spp is done by using optochin, bacitracin trimethoprim-sulfamethoxazole discs, bile aesculin agar and CAMP test [44]. Interpretation of *Streptococcus* identification tests is shown in table below.

Table 1; Basic identification tests for *Streptococcus* spp pathogens [44].

Streptococcus spp	Group	Hemolysis	Optochin	Bacitracin	SXT	Bile aesculin	CAMP test
S. pyogenes	A	beta	X	√	X	XX	XX
S. agalactiae	B	beta	X	X	X	XX	√√
S. pneumoniae	NA	alpha	√	d	√	XX	XX
Enterococcus faecalis	D	alpha	X	X	X	√√	XX

Key; X=Not sensitive, √=Sensitive, √√=Positive, XX=Negative and d=differential reactions

Principle of bile aesculin test for identification of *E. faecalis*

Enterococcus spp grows in 40% bile and are capable of hydrolyzing aesculin in the medium resulting to blackening of agar in test tube.

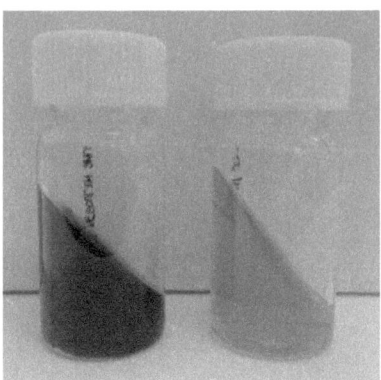

Figure 13: Bile aesculin test. Positive (left) and negative (right).

CAMP test

It is used for identification and confirmation of group B streptococcus spp., such as *S. agalactiae* which produces "CAMP factor" in the presence of beta hemolytic *S. aureus* ATCC 25923 which produces "beta-hemolysin" enzyme. When lines of these species are streaked perpendicular to each close enough but not touching one another, they synergize to increase hemolysis of the sheep blood in agar, making an arrow head shape [15, 79].

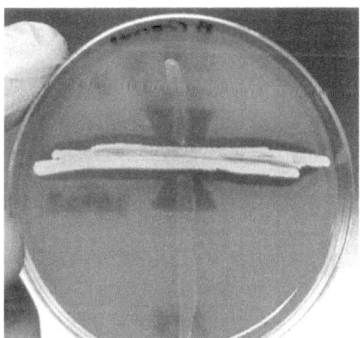

Figure 14: Arrow heads of *S. agalactiae* above and below the horizontally inoculated *S. aureus* (Source: Wikipedia the free encyclopedia, CAMP test)

Identification of gram negative bacteria

At least five biochemical identification tests can be employed for identification of about all common pathogens causing human infectious diseases in the family *Enterobacteriaceae*. These tests are oxidase test, triple sugar iron (TSI) test agar, sulfur indole motility (SIM) test agar, Simon's citrate test agar and urease test agar [16].

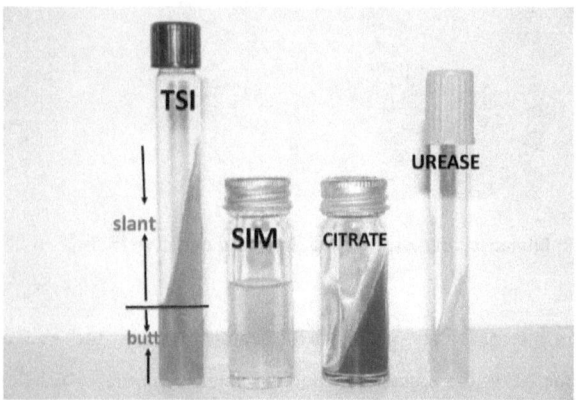

Figure 15: Set of biochemical identification tests for gram negative bacteria. TSI test, SIM test, Simmon's citrate test and Urease test (from left to right).

Oxidase test

This test is used for identification of none lactose fermenting gram negative bacteria, however some gram positive bacteria are also positive for this test. Bacteria produces cytochrome c oxidase enzyme which reduces tetramethyl-p-phenylene diamine dihydrochloride substrate in the white paper test into deep purple color. *Pseudomonas*, *Neisseria* and *Vibrio* spp., are positive for this test [79].

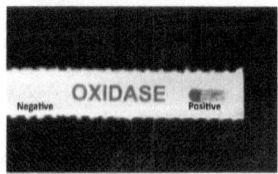

Figure 16: Oxidase test strip, negative on the left hand side and positive on the right hand side.

TSI test

This test detects the ability of bacteria to ferment sugars (glucose, sucrose and lactose), produce carbon dioxide (CO_2) gas and production of hydrogen sulfide (H_2S). Fermentation of sugars shift agar's Ph into acidic which is indicated by changing color from red to yellow with phenol red indicator. Production of H_2S is indicated by blackening of the medium by ferrous sulfate indicator. Production of gas is observed by the presence of cracks of gas bubbles in the medium.

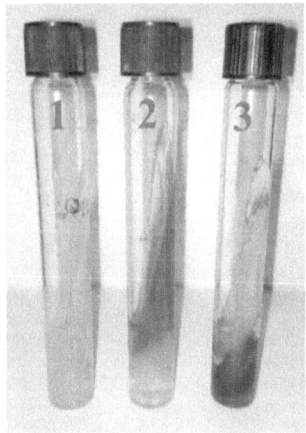

Figure 17; Inoculated TSI tests. 1. Slant-Acid/Butt-Acid, gas-positive and sulfur-negative. 2. Slant-Alkali/Butt-Acid, gas-negative and sulfur-negative. 3. Slant-Acid/Butt-Acid, gas-positive and sulfur-positive.

Sulfur-indole-motility (SIM) test

This test detects bacteria's ability to produce H_2S, indole and motility. Principle of H_2S production, refer TSI test. Bacteria produces tryptophanase enzymes which convert tryptophan into indole, upon addition of Kovac's reagent indole give reddish color on top of the medium. Motility is detected by clear medium turning into turbidity after inoculation and incubation of test bacteria.

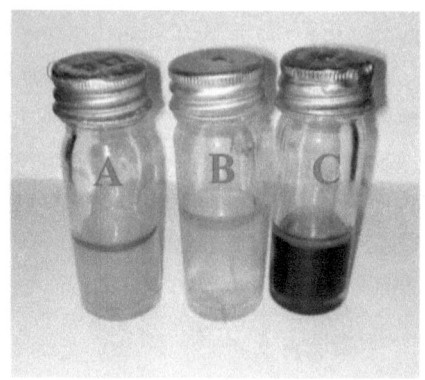

Figure 18; Inoculated SIM tests. (A). Sulfur-negative, Indole-positive and Motility-positive. (B). Sulfur-negative, Indole-negative and Motility-negative. (C). Sulfur-positive, Indole-negative and Motility-positive.

Simmons citrate test

The test detects ability of bacteria to utilize citrate as the core source of energy as carbon and inorganic ammonium salts. Bacteria produces citrate-permease enzyme which metabolize citrate while breaking down ammonium salts to ammonia increasing alkalinity of the medium turning the color of medium from green to blue in the presence of bromothymol blue indicator [44].

Urease test

Those bacteria producing urease enzyme they break down urea in the medium into ammonia and CO_2. Ammonia alkalinize the medium increasing its Ph that can be indicated by color change of phenol red indicator from light yellow to pinkish [80].

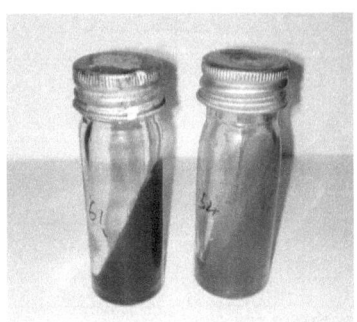

Figure 19; Simmons citrate positive test (left) and urease positive test (right).

Interpretation of biochemical identification tests

A combination of biochemical test results is required to come into a conclusion of the bacterial species isolated. For the specimens collected from none sterile sites for example stool specimen, the identified bacteria should be determined if it is normal GIT flora or pathogen, and if it is a pathogen, then antimicrobial susceptibility testing is done to guide rational therapy of the patient.

Table 2; Interpretation of common biochemical identification tests for medically important Gram negative bacteria to species level [15, 16, 44].

Species	TSI/KIA Medium			SIM Medium		SIM/TSI	Citrate	Urease	Oxidase
	Slope	But t	Gas	Indole	Motility	H₂S			
Escherichia coli	Y	Y	+	+	+	-	-	-	-
Shigella spp	R	Y	-	d	-	-	-	-	-
Salmonella typhi	R	Y	-	-	+	+	-	-	-
Salmonella paratyphi-A	R	Y	+	-	+	-	-	-	-
Salmonella typhimariam	R	Y	d	-	+	+	d	+	-
Citrobacter freundii	R/Y	Y	+	-	+	d	+	d	-
Citrobacter koseri	Y	Y	+	+	+	+	+	-	-
Klebsiella pneumoniae	Y	Y	+	-	-	-	+	+	-
Klebsiella oxytoca	Y	Y	+	+	-	-	+	+	-
Enterobacter aerogenes	Y	Y	+	-	+	-	+	-	-
Enterobacter cloacae	Y	Y	+	-	+	-	+	+	d

Serratia marcescens	R/Y	Y	d	-	+	-	+	d	-
Proteus vulgaris	R	Y	d	+	+	+	d	+	-
Proteus mirabilis	R	Y	+	-	+	+	+	+	-
Providencia spp	R	Y	d	+	+	-	+	d	-
Morganella morganii	R	Y	d	+	+	-	-	+	-
Yersinia enterocolitica	R	Y	-	d	+	-	-	+	-
Vibrio cholerae	R	Y	-	+	+	-	d	-	+
Aeromonas hydrophilia	Y	Y	+	+	+	-	+	-	+
Pseudomonas aeruginosa	R	R	-	-	+	-	+	d	+
Acinetobacter spp	R	R	-	-	-	-	+	-	-

KEY: d=differential, it can be positive or negative

Analytical profile index (API) system

API stands for Analytical Profile Index is a commercial standardized system for identification of different bacteria including Enterobacteriaceae, other Gram-negative rods and Gram-positive bacteria [81]. It was discovered by Pierre Janin in 1970s. There are two API systems namely, API-20E/NE and API-Staph. API-20E/NE for identification of Enterobacteriaceae and non-Enterobacteriaceae Gram-negative bacteria. API-Staph for identification of Gram-positive bacteria which are Staphylococci, Micrococci and other related bacteria.

The test strips of API system consist of wells which contains dehydrated substrates. Substrates detect enzymatic products of carbohydrates fermentation and catabolism of amino acid or proteins from inoculated bacteria [81]. Wells on API strips system are rehydrated by homogenous bacterial suspension in 0.85% sterile saline, and then the strips are incubated at 36°C ± 2°C for 18-24 hours [81]. During incubation, enzyme-substrate reactions produces color changes that are either spontaneous or revealed by the addition of reagents [81]. For example, pH indicator changes color when pH within the well decreases after carbohydrates are fermented.

All positive and negative test results are compiled to obtain a profile number, and the identification is obtained by referring to the Analytical Profile Index or using the identification software [81].

API 20 E after incubation...Positive results for all tests :

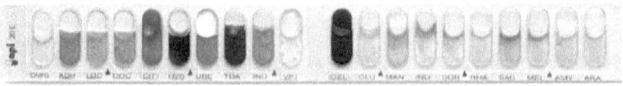

API 20 E after incubation...Negative results for all tests :

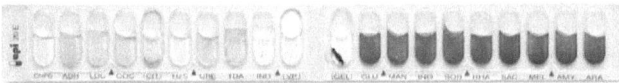

Figure 20: API 20E system for identification of Enterobacteriaceae showing positive results (top) negative results (bottom). (Source: Jody Riley, 2016. Bacteria identification)

The advantage of API system over conventional biochemical identification tests, it has a wide number of biochemical tests therefore increasing the identification range of bacteria. However its disadvantages over conventional biochemical Identification tests, is the use of online softwares for interpretation of profile numbers to identify isolates to their species levels. In most low and middle income countries (LMICs), availability of reliable internet services is still a big challenge. Further, online database for identifcations of bacteria require frequently updates.

153

Antimicrobial susceptibility testing
Introduction

Disc diffusion technique is a simple method for antibiotic susceptibility testing which may be performed in laboratory settings with limited resources. Bacteria suspensions equivalent to 0.5McFarland turbidity stand solution are swabbed onto agar base for antimicrobial disc diffusion susceptibility testing. Within 15 minutes, antibiotic specific antibiotic discs are then seeded and plates are aerobically incubated at 37 degree Celsius for 18-24 hours. Zones of inhibitions are then interpreted as sensitive or intermediate or resistant according to international standard guidelines such as Clinical and Laboratory Standard Institute (CLSI) or European Committee on Antimicrobial Susceptibility Testing (EUCAST).

AST can be done through numbers of techniques; E test, broth/agar micro dilution and disc diffusion [82, 83]. The named techniques are grouped into qualitative and quantitative methods [84]. Qualitative method tells whether bacteria is sensitive or resistant to antibiotic agent only for example disc diffusion technique while quantitative method tells even the quantity of antibiotic the bacteria is sensitive to, for example E test and broth/agar micro dilution techniques [84]. In this chapter, disc diffusion technique and agar micro dilution technique will be discussed as because these techniques are cost effective and they can be performed under resources limited bacteriology laboratory.

Disc diffusion technique

Specific concentration of an antimicrobial agent in 6 mm circular disc is allowed to diffuse into solid culture medium where it is seeded where specific test bacteria suspension was evenly swabbed over the entire medium [82, 83]. After 18 to 24 hours of incubation, zones of inhibitions of antimicrobial discs are determined and interpreted for susceptibility results [82, 83]. But suspension of test bacteria for making inoculation on susceptibility culture plates should be standardized by the use of 0.5% McFarland turbidity standard solution. Too thick suspension will result to false reduced zones of inhibitions while too thin suspension will results to false increased zones of inhibitions. The impact of this error in making suspension is in vitro susceptibility pattern will not give the same results as in vivo treatment expected outcome.

Some of antimicrobial agents to be set for susceptibility testing are narrow spectrum while others are broad spectrum [85, 86]. Selection of antimicrobial discs should be done considering specificity of the discs; narrow spectrum, either for gram negative or gram positive bacteria only (narrow range of activity) for example vancomycin for *Staphylococcus* spp and broad spectrum, for both gram negative and gram positive bacteria (broad range of activity) for example gentamicin and ciprofloxacin [85, 87]. Selection of antimicrobial agents with specific to gram reaction of the bacteria is shown in the table 1. Interpretation of zones of inhibitions; sensitive, intermediate or resistant is shown in table 2.

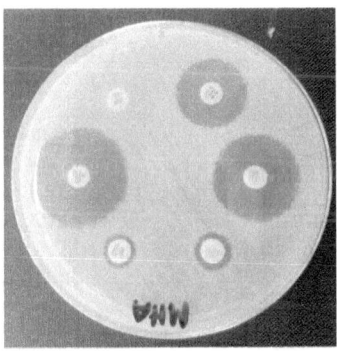

Figure 1; Antimicrobial susceptibility testing by disk diffusion technique on Muller Hintoin agar (MHA)

Table 1: Basic sets of antibiotics for routine susceptibility testing for specific isolated bacteria species

Staphylococcus/Streptoc occus/Enterococcus species	Enterobacteriaceae	Acinetobacter spp	Pseudomonas spp
Gentamicin	Ampicillin	Amikacin	Piperacillin
Azithromycin	Amikacin	Gentamicin	Piperacillin-tazobactam
Tetracycline	Amoxycillin-clavulanate	Tetracycline	Ceftazidime
Ciprofloxacin	Azithromycin	Ciprofloxacin	Cefepime
Nitrofurantoin (isolates from urine ONLY)	Piperacillin-tazobactam	Trimethoprim-sulfamethoxazole	Gentamicin
Clindamycin	Cefepime	Ceftazidime	Amikacin
Trimethoprim-sulfamethoxazole	Cefotaxime	Ceftriaxone	Ciprofloxacin
Vancomycin	Ceftriaxone	Imipenem	Imipenem
Cefoxitin (for *S. aureus* ONLY)	Cefoxitin	Meropenem	Meropenem
Linezolid	Ceftazidime		
	Cefpodoxime		
	Gentamicin		
	Ciprofloxacin		
	Tetracycline		
	Imipenem		
	Meropenem		
	Nitrofurantoin (for urine isolates ONLY)		
	Trimethoprim-sulfamethoxazole		

Table 2: Interpretation of zone diameter breakpoints for antibiotics susceptibility testing

Antimicrobial agent for Enterobacteriaceae	Disk content	Zone diameter breakpoints (mm)		
		S	I	R
Ampicillin	10µg	≥17	14-16	≤13
Amikacin	30µg	≥17	15-16	≤14
Amoxycillin-clavulanate	20/10µg	≥18	14-17	≤13
Azithromycin	15µg	≥13	-	≤12
Piperacillin-tazobactam	100/10µg	≥21	18-20	≤17
Cefepime	30µg	≥25	-	≤18
Cefotaxime	30µg	≥26	23-25	≤22
Ceftriaxone	30µg	≥23	20-22	≤19
Cefoxitin	30µg	≥18	15-17	≤14
Ceftazidime	30µg	≥21	18-20	≤17
Cefpodoxime	10µg	≥21	18-20	≤17
Gentamicin	10µg	≥15	13-14	≤12
Ciprofloxacin	5µg	≥21	16-20	≤15
Tetracycline	30µg	≥15	12-14	≤11
Trimethoprim-sulfamethoxazole	1.25/23.75µg	≥16	11-15	≤10
Imipenem	10µg	≥23	20-22	≤19
Meropenem	10µg	≥23	20-22	≤19
Nitrofurantoin	300µg	≥17	15-16	≤14
Antimicrobial agents for *Staphylococcus/Streptococcus/Enterococcus* species				
Gentamicin**	10µg	≥15	13-14	≤12
Azithromycin	15µg	≥18	14-17	≤13
Erythromycin	15µg			
Staphylococcus & *Enterococcus* spp		≥23	14-22	≤13
Streptococcus spp		≥21	16-20	≤15
Tetracycline	30µg			
Staphylococcus & *Enterococcus* spp		≥19	15-18	≤14
Streptococcus spp		≥28	25-27	≤24
Ciprofloxacin	5µg	≥21	16-20	≤15
Nitrofurantoin (*Staphylococcus* and *Enterococcus* spp., isolated from urine)	300µg	≥17	15-16	≤14
Clindamycin**	2µg			
Staphylococcus spp		≥21	15-20	≤14
Streptococcus spp		≥19	16-18	≤15
Trimethoprim-sulfamethoxazole**	1.25/23.75µg			
Staphylococcus spp		≥16	11-15	≤10
Streptococcus spp		≥19	16-18	≤15
Vancomycin***	30µg			
Enterococcus spp		≥17	15-16	≤14
Streptococcus spp		≥17	-	-
Cefoxitin (for *S. aureus* ONLY)	30µg	≥22	-	≤21
Ampicillin****	10µg	≥17	-	≤16

	30µg			
Linezolid	30µg			
Staphylococcus spp		≥21	-	≤20
Enterococcus spp		≥23	21-22	≤20
Streptococcus spp		≥21	-	-
Antimicrobial agents for *Acinetobacter* spp & *Pseudomonas* spp				
Amikacin	30µg	≥17	15-16	≤14
Piperacillin	100µg			
Acinetobacter spp		≥21	18-20	≤17
Pseudomonas spp		≥21	15-20	≤14
Piperacillin-tazobactam	100/10µg			
Acinetobacter spp		≥21	18-20	≤17
Pseudomonas spp		≥21	15-20	≤14
Gentamicin	10µg	≥15	13-14	≤12
Tetracycline (*Acinetobacter* spp ONLY)	30µg	≥15	12-14	≤11
Ciprofloxacin	5µg	≥21	16-20	≤15
Trimethoprim-sulfamethoxazole (*Acinetobacter* spp ONLY)	µg	≥16	11-15	≤10
Ceftazidime	30µg	≥18	15-17	≤14
Ceftriaxone	30µg	≥21	14-20	≤13
Imipenem	10µg			
Acinetobacter spp		≥22	19-21	≤18
Pseudomonas spp		≥19	16-18	≤15
Meropenem	10µg			
Acinetobacter spp		≥18	15-17	≤14
Pseudomonas spp		≥19	16-18	≤15
Cefepime	10µg	≥18	15-17	≤14

*For *Salmonella* spp., and *Shigella* spp., may appear active in-vitro but are not effective clinically and should not be reported.

**For *Enterococcus* spp., may appear active in-vitro but are not effective clinically and should not be reported.

***No interpretation of zones for *S. aureus*

****For *Enterococcus* spp., ONLY.

Source: CLSI (2018). Performance standards for antimicrobial susceptibility testing, M100, 28th Edition

Note: CLSI updates zone diameter breakpoints at-least in every year, laboratory should keep updated with every edition released for reliability of antibiotics susceptibility results

Agar micro dilution technique

This is a semi quantitative method which measures the lowest/minimum inhibitory concentration (MIC) of antimicrobial agent capable to inhibit microbes' growth on nutrient agar [88]. Muller Hinton agar (MHA) plates are supplemented with different concentrations of antimicrobial agents, for example four types of MHA are made whereby each type is supplemented with specific concentration of antimicrobial agent, which is 2µg/ml cefotaxime, 4µg/ml cefotaxime, 8µg/ml cefotaxime and 16µg/ml cefotaxime. Test bacteria are sub-cultured onto both MHA plate, incubated for 18 to 24 hours. Interpretation of this technique is, bacteria is resistant to antimicrobial agent if grown in all concentrations of cefotaxime supplemented in MHA or bacteria is sensitive to antimicrobial agent if inhibited to grow on certain concentration(s) on MHA. The lowest concentration to inhibit bacteria growth is referred to as minimum inhibitory concentration and it is exact amount of antibiotic should be given to specific patient [88, 89]. Antibiotics for injection can be used for this technique, calculated to specific concentrations of interests.

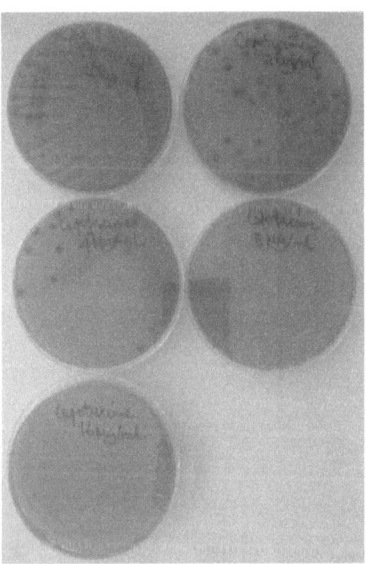

Figure 21: Agar microdilution test. MacConkey agar plates supplemented with cefotaxime of different concentrations; 1µg/ml (top left), 2µg/ml (top right), 4µg/ml (middle left), 8µg/ml

(middle right) and 16µg/ml (bottom left). Bacteria was inhibited to grow on 8µg/ml and 16µg/ml plates, therefore MIC is 8µg/ml.

Advantage of agar micro dilution technique are, it tells susceptibility of bacteria with exact lowest concentration of antimicrobial agent (minimum inhibitory concentration) and it is cost effective as even ten test bacteria can be sub-cultured onto one MHA plate as only growth is determined [88].

Broth micro-dilution technique

This semi-quantitative method measures the lowest (minimum) concentration of specific antimicrobial agent able to inhibit visible bacterial growth on broth media. Therefore it determines the minimum inhibitory concentration (MIC) of antimicrobial agents on broth media. Microbes are inoculated into broth tubes or microtiter plates containing antimicrobial agents at an increased concentrations, usually doubling dilutions for example 1, 2, 4, 8, 16 and 32 µg/ml. Bacterial suspension is supposed to be between 1×10^5 CFU/ml and 5×10^5 CFU/ml. then, tubes or microtiter plates are incubated aerobically at 35-37^{0}C for 16-24 hours. After incubation, growth is assessed by either visually or by the aid of automated readers. The minimum concentration of antimicrobial agent that inhibited growth represent the MIC [88, 90].

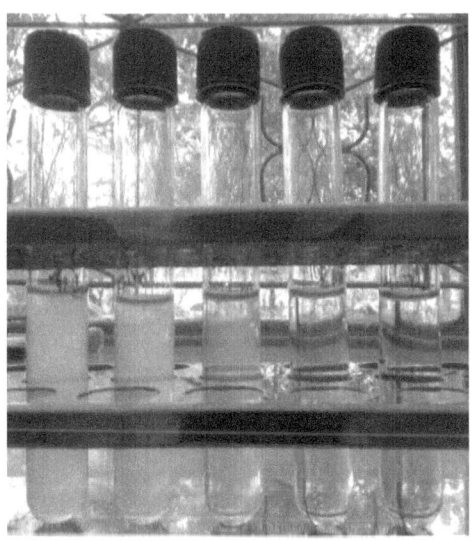

Figure 22: Broth microdilution test. Inoculated tubes with nutrient broth containing cefotaxime; 1µg/ml, 2µg/ml, 4µg/ml, 8µg/ml and 16µg/ml (from left to right). Third (8µg/ml) and fourth (16µg/ml) tubes are visible clear, therefore MIC is 8µg/ml.

Epsilometer test (E-test) technique

These non-porous plastic carrier strips (5mm × 60mm) consist of predefined, continuous and exponential gradient of antimicrobial concentrations immobilized along the strip. The test provides direct quantity of antimicrobial concentration an organism is susceptible. The test applies both microdilution and diffusion of antimicrobial agent on single testing strip. Antimicrobial agent from test strip diffuses into agar medium while establishing antimicrobial concentration gradient on medium. Inoculated plates are incubated at 37^{0}C for 24 hours. After incubation, a symmetrical inhibition ellipse (drop-shaped zone of inhibition) is produced intersecting test strip at the minimum inhibitory concentration (MIC) [91, 92].

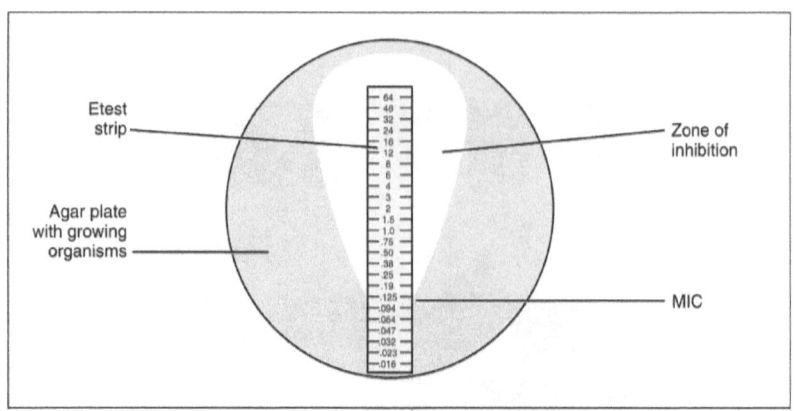

Figure 23: E-test showing drop-like zone of inhibition and MIC (Source: Principles of Antimicrobial Chemotherapy/Basicmedical Key).

VITEK 2 system: identification and antibiotic susceptibility testing

Rapid and accurate isolation, identification and antibiotic susceptibility testing of infectious bacteria (especially during this era of increasing multi-drug resistant bacteria) is the key to providing the right information for targeted clinical response for better patients' outcomes [93]. Thus, technology is advancing from conventional culture and susceptibility testing which takes a minimum of 72 hours to the VITEK 2 system which provides final results in a less than 48 hours.

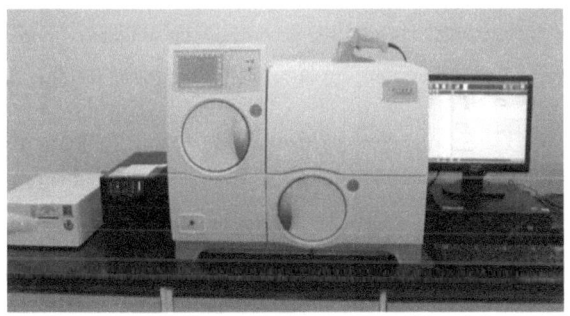

Figure 24: VITEK 2 Compact system (Source: Badawy *et al.*, 2013 [94])

The VITEK 2 system is an automated system which identifies bacteria by using fluorogenic methodology and test their susceptibility patterns by using turbidimetric method on a 64 well reagent (test) card that is barcoded [95, 96]. The VITEK 2 system is available in three formats: VITEK 2 compact, VITEK 2, and VITEK 2 XL. The VITEK 2 compact is provided with wide application of industrial Bacteriology (Microbiology) laboratories but the VITEK 2 and VITEK 2 XL are applicable for clinical Bacteriology (Microbiology) laboratories [95, 96]. There are four reagent (test) cards (kits) which are categorized into two major groups: two identification (ID-GN (Gram-negative bacillus identification) and ID-GP (Gram-positive cocci identification)) and two antibiotic susceptibility testing (AST-GN (Gram-negative susceptibility) and AST-GP (Gram-positive susceptibility)) cards [95, 96]. ID-GN card identifies 154 species of Enterobacteriaceae and other selected non-fermenting Gram-negative bacilli [95, 96]. The ID-GP card identifies 124 species of staphylococci, streptococci, enterococci and other selected Gram-positive spore forming bacteria [95, 96]. For AST, the VITEK 2 system provides results in minimum inhibitory concentration (MIC) within 5 to 8 hours [93].

Preparation of suspension for bacteria ID and AST

Sufficient number of colonies from pure and fresh culture (age of culture: ≤ 24 hours old) are transferred in a tube with at least 3 ml of 0.45 - 0.50% sterile saline by using sterile swab or applicator stick or disposable loop [95]. Colonies are then suspended making a homogenous suspension with a density equivalent to 0.50 – 0.63 McFarland standard using the DensiCHEK Plus or visible comparison with in-house made or commercial 0.5 McFarland standard tube [95]. Any deviation of the turbidity is adjusted accordingly by addition of more bacteria colonies for too thin turbidity or addition of more sterile saline for too thick turbidity.

Note: for AST, 145ul of the 0.50 – 0.63 turbidity suspension prepared is added into another tube of 3 ml of 0.45 – 0.50% sterile saline for AST-GN cards, or 280ul of the suspension for AST-GP cards [96].

Inoculation and incubation of cards

Test tubes containing suspended bacteria and their corresponding ID or AST cards are placed on slots of the special rack known as cassette [95]. These cassettes can accommodate from 10 to 15 tests. Then, the cassette is placed either manually or automatically into a vacuum chamber of the VITEK 2 system which transfers bacteria suspension by vacuum into micro-channels to fill all wells of the cards [95]. Transfer tubes are cut off and sealed automatically in the system, and then the cards are loaded into carousel incubator which can accommodate between 30 and 60 cards at a time. Incubation temperature of the carousel incubator is 35.5 ± 1.0⯑C [95].

ID results

For bacteria ID, based on the calculated confidence interval, the VITEK 2 system displays one of the four types of results: consistent result (correct identification), inconsistent result (strains of low discrimination, review of results is required), unknown phenotype (proposed strain is different with reference) and phenotype not in database (no identification) [93, 97].

Culture of *Mycobacterium tuberculosis* complex (MTBC)

Microscopic diagnosis of AFB is regarded as preliminary diagnosis as to about 50% of AFB culture positive may become smear negative which were made directly from the specimens. Therefore, culture diagnosis of AFB infection plays significant role in diagnosis of TB. Currently, different culture media are in use, liquid and solid. Example of solid culture media is egg-based Lowenstein-Jensen (LT) agar and liquid culture media are BACTEC 460 TB system, MB Redox tube system and BACTEC MGIT 960 system. Laboratory procedures for the diagnosis of TB should be conducted in Biosafety level 2 laboratory with negative pressure and sufficient ventilation system [98].

Liquid culture on Mycobacteria Growth Indicator Tube, BACTEC MGIT 960 system

The purpose of this technique is to amplify the number of Mycobacterium tuberculosis (MTB) organisms in a sample using a nutritious liquid culture media (MGIT) and for a detection of positive sample in a short period of time [99].

While nutritious-rich media allows the multiplication of Mycobacteria, other contaminating bacteria are inhibited by cocktail of antibiotics. As oxygen saturation decreases in the tube, proportionally number of Mycobacteria cells multiply. Multiplied Mycobacteria are indicated by fluorescence which is detected by MGIT instrument using UV light and complex computer algorithms [99]. The following procedures should be used for preparation of specimens to be inoculated into MGIT tubes [98].

Required materials for preparation of sputum samples for BACTEC MGIT 960 system

- Disposable 50 ml Falcon tubes
- Sterile NaOH-NALC-sodium citrate solution (a mixture of 4% NaOH and 2.9% sodium citrate solution)
- Commercially or laboratory prepared sterile phosphate buffer pH 6.8 (0.067M).
- Centrifuge machine (capacity: 3000-3500 rpm)
- Vortex mixer or shaker
- Timer
- Pasteur pipettes

Procedures for preparation of sputum samples for BACTEC MGIT 960 system

- Samples should be transferred into 50ml falcon tubes (centrifuge tubes if were not collected in these kind of tubes)
- Equal volume of NaOH-NALC-sodium citrate solution is added into 50ml falcon tubes containing specimens
- Gently mix specimen with NaOH-NALC-sodium citrate solution in tubes by vortex mixer or shake or by hand for about 15-30 seconds.
- Tubes should be let stand for 15-25 minutes, gently mix the samples after every 5-10 minutes
- At the end of 15-25 minutes specimen supposed to be completely liquefied but if still mucoid, a small quantity of NALC powder (30-35 grams) should be added directly to the specimen tube
- After liquefied, phosphate buffer (pH 6.8) is added up to the top ring on the sample tubes and then mixed well (sterile water is not a suitable alternative for the phosphate buffer)
- Sample tubes are then centrifuged at 3000 rpm or more for 15-20 minutes. Use of refrigerated centrifugation is known to increase recovery of mycobacteria)
- Tubes are allowed to sit for 5 minutes to allow aerosols to settle.
- Then supernatant is carefully discarded into a suitable container containing mycobactericidal disinfectant.
- The sediment is re-suspended by adding a small quantity (1-2 ml) of phosphate buffer (pH 6.8)
- Re-suspended pellet are used for making smears and for inoculation of MGIT tubes

Inoculation of MGIT tubes

Well mixed sediments of sputum specimen (0.5ml each) is inoculated into 7ml MGIT tubes containing 0.8ml mixture of cocktail antibiotics (PANTA)/growth supplement (OADC). Antibiotics cocktail in PANTA include polymyxin B, amphotericin B, nalidixic acid, trimethoprim, and azlocillin [100]. Growth supplements in OADC are oleic acid, albumin from bovine, dextrose, catalase [100]. Tubes are tightly recapped and mixed gently, then entered into MGIT instrument as soon as possible. The MGIT instrument incubates and monitor tubes in stations automatically and continuously until signals "POSITIVE" (any time) or "NEGATIVE" (after 42 days of incubation) [99].

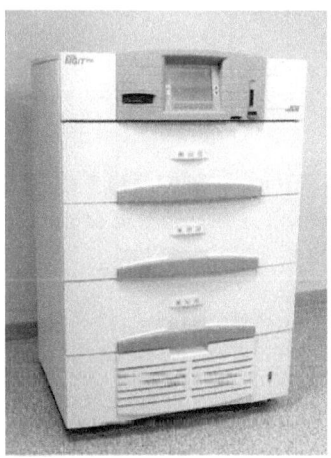

Figure 25: Becton Dickinson BACTEC MGIT (Source: New Life Scientific Inc, US)

Susceptibility testing using BACTEC MGIT 960 system

For susceptibility testing of positive specimens, two MGIT tubes are prepared, one labeled control (C) and another labeled test (T). These tubes should also be labeled with specimen given laboratory number. All tubes are inoculated with test culture (from previous MGIT tube which displayed and confirmed positive), but one tube (T) is added with known and recommended concentration of antimycobacterial drug and mixed well. These tubes are then incubated into BACTEC MGIT 960 system. If drug is effective, decreased fluorescence in tube T and increased fluorescence in tube C will be detected [98].

Solid culture on Lowenstein-Jensen media (LJ media)

Lowenstein-Jensen (LJ) agar is the selective medium which is used for the cultivation and isolation of Mycobacteria. LJ media was named after Lowenstein who incorporated congo-red and malachite green to inhibit nonmycobacteria and Jensen who removed congo-red but uses a moderate of malachite green to prevent nonmycobacteria. The present formulation, egg-based medium, was formulated during Jensen's modification. Other formulations of LJ media are

167

potato flour, L-Asparagine, monopotassium phosphate, magnesium citrate, malachite green, magnesium sulfate, glycerol and egg suspension [101].

L-Asparagine and potato flour provides required nitrogen and vitamins for in vitro growth of Mycobacteria. Monopotassium phosphate and magnesium sulfate facilitates growth and provides favorable pH for growth of Mycobacteria. Malachite green, support the selective nature of LJ media by inhibiting nonmycobacteria from growing on this media. During their growth, Mycobacteria metabolize using fatty acids and protein from egg suspension. Also, when heated, coagulating egg albumin provides a solid surface for inoculation. Glycerol is a carbon source and favors the growth of Mycobacteria of the human type than the bovine type [101].

Preparation of sputum for culture on LJ media

- In centrifuge tubes, about 2-5ml of sputum sample is added following addition of equal volume of 4% NaOH.
- Tubes are screw capped and then mixture of sputum samples and 4% NaOH are mixed well by vortex mixer or shaker to digest mucus from sputum samples.
- Mixed samples are allowed to stand for 15 minutes at room temperature.
- Then, phosphate buffer is added to fill the tubes (e.g. to the 50-ml mark if falcon tubes are used).
- Following centrifugation of samples at 3000g for 15 minutes.
- Carefully, supernatant is discarded into a discard can containing 5% phenol or other mycobacterial disinfectant.
- Deposits are re-suspended using phosphate buffer (about 0.3 ml) following gently mixing.
- Re-suspended deposits are then inoculated on two slopes of egg-based LJ media labelled with the laboratory given numbers.
- Each LJ medium is inoculated with 3–4 drops of appropriate sample.
- One drop of sample should be smeared on clean, greasy free slide, labeled with laboratory given number, for microscopic examination after heat fixed and stained.

Tubes of LJ media are incubated upright at 37⁰C (±1⁰C) and examined and recorded weekly until become positive or till week 8. When observing and reading of culture tubes they should be tightened. Colonies of *M. tuberculosis* are usually dry, buff-colored, and very distinctive [99].

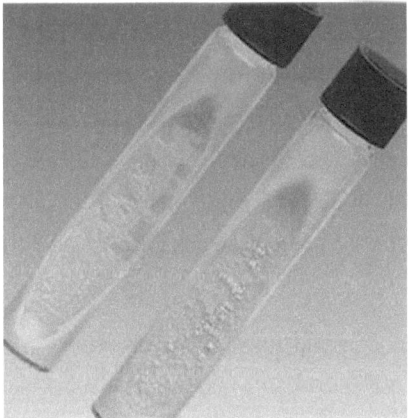

Figure 26: Positive growth of Mycobacteria on LJ media (Source: Fisher Scientific, Thermo Scientific Remel™ Lowenstein-Jensen Medium (LJ))

TB diagnosis by Gene Xpert MTB/RIF assay

WHO is recommending on the use of Xpert MTB/RIF as the initial diagnostic test in adults and children suspected of having MDR-TB or HIV-associated TB rather than conventional microscopy, culture and DST. Moreover, Xpert MTB/RIF is recommended when further testing of smear-negative specimens is necessary in adults suspected of having TB who are not at risk of MDR-TB or HIV-associated TB. Also, WHO is recommending the use of Xpert MTB/RIF in diagnosis of extra pulmonary TB with non-sputum specimens such as cerebrospinal fluid (CSF) specimens from patients suspected of having TB meningitis from its urgency of rapid diagnosis. Sensitivity of Xpert MTB/RIF in detection of TB meningitis is 79.5% using culture as a gold standard. Other homogenized non-sputum samples can be used for the diagnosis of extra-pulmonary TB [102].

Gene Xpert MTB/RIF assay (Xpert MTB/RIF) principally based on nucleic acid amplification (NAA) to simultaneously detect DNA of Mycobacterium tuberculosis complex (MTBC) and rifampin resistance (RIF) (i.e. mutation of the *rpo*B gene, 81 bp) within 2 hours. Standard culture can take 2-6 weeks for MTBC to grow adding another 3 weeks for conventional drug susceptibility. Xpert MTB/RIF is integrated with automatic sample processing, and amplification and detection of the target sequences of nucleic acid. The Xpert MTB/RIF probes can differentiate mutations associated with rifampicin resistance from the conserved wild-type sequence [103].

Procedures of sputum samples for Xpert MTB/RIF assay

Raw and direct sputum or decontaminated and concentrated sputum (refer procedures prior to solid culture) samples can be used.

- Xpert MTB/RIF sample reagent is mixed with sputum in specimen container (2:1 volume by volume).
- Mixture of reagent and sputum sample is mixed well and allowed to stand for not less than 15 minutes at room temperature.
- Xpert MTB/RIF cartilages are labeled with laboratory given numbers of specific specimens (NOTE: do not label or attach ID label on 2D barcode on the cartilage).

- Then aspirate liquefied samples from specimen containers into appropriately labeled Xpert MTB/RIF cartilages using sterile pasteur pipettes provided.
- Xpert MTB/RIF cartilages lids should be closed firmly.
- Xpert MTB/RIF cartilages are transferred into open slots/ports of the Xpert MTB/RIF analyzer and doors are closed.
- Testing of samples by Xpert MTB/RIF analyzer should start within 30 minutes.

For insufficient samples no further processing is recommended and for excess liquefied samples can be refrigerated at 2-8⁰C for 12 hours because they may be used in-case of invalid results.

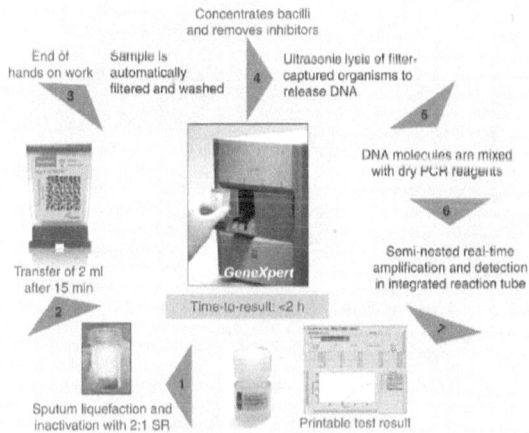

Figure 27: Assay procedures of sputum samples for Xpert MTB/RIF machine [104]

Interpretation of Xpert MTB/RIF assay results

On completion of sample testing, Xpert MTB/RIF assay will display "MTBC detected" or "MTB not detected" and sometimes "INVALID". If MTB detected, RIF resistance will be stated either detected, not detected or indeterminate. All samples given "INVALID" results should be repeated [103].

171

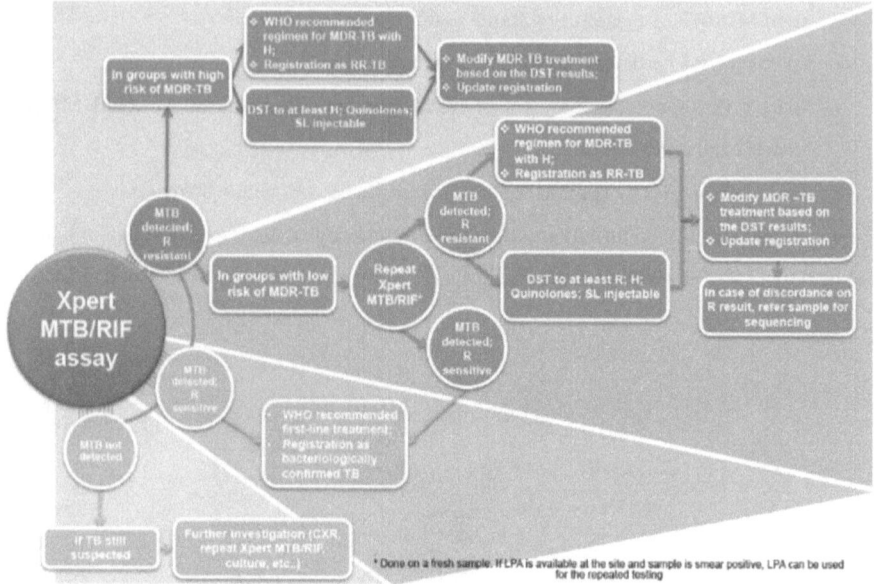

Figure 28: Interpretation of Xpert MTB/RIF results and way forward for each result (Source: WHO, Xpert MTB/RIF implementation manual)

Phenotypic detection of multi-drug resistant (MDR) bacteria
Introduction

Multi-drug resistant bacteria are serious global public health concerns with adverse negative impact to patients' managements. The impact is serious in low and middle income countries where technology is lagging behind. Increased healthcare costs, days of hospitalization, morbidity and mortality are the major challenges of multi-drug resistant infections. Regardless of limited methodologies for detection of multi-drug resistant bacteria, still there are cost-effective and reliable phenotypic techniques which can be applied and used in any bacteriology laboratory. Phenotypic techniques for detection of multi-drug resistant bacteria are significant for patients' management and provision of data for global fight against multi-drug resistance.

Researchers and international standards such as Clinical and Laboratory Standard Institute (CLSI) have recommended some phenotypic techniques to detect AMR [105]. Clinical laboratories in low and middle income countries may adopt these techniques to detect AMR infections which will have great impact on treatment, prevention and control of infectious diseases. With added advantage, it will make availability of information on AMR from these countries which will be very useful for Microbiologists, Molecular epidemiologists and Clinicians in the fight against antibiotics resistant "priority pathogens".

Phenotypic detection of antibiotics resistant "priority pathogens" can be achieved when performing routine antibiotics susceptibility testing. Bacteria resistance to certain class of antibiotics or phenotypic patterns of zones of inhibitions when two or three antibiotics discs are arranged edge to edge by one another. Different molecular epidemiological studies have been appreciated antimicrobial resistance phenotypes in predicting possible resistant genes harbored by specific bacteria. In this laboratory guidebook; induced clindamycin resistance, methicillin resistance *Staphylococcus aureus* (MRSA), Amp-C beta lactamase, extended spectrum beta lactamase (ESBL) and carbapenemase will be explained in brief.

Induced clindamycin resistance

Detection of Inducible clindamycin resistance is therefore phenotypically detected by disk diffusion technique using D-test of which 2µg clindamycin and 15µg erythromycin are placed between 15 and 20 mm apart. Diffusion of erythromycin towards erythromycin is inducing production of erythromycin inducible methylase from *S. aureus* around the two antibiotics discs making a flattering zone of inhibition ("D" shape) of clindamycin on side of erythromycin [106].

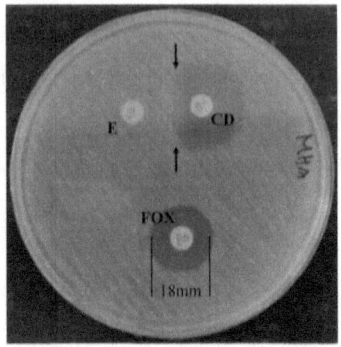

Figure 29: *S. aureus* **co-production of beta-lactamase enzyme (MRSA) and erythromycin inducible methylase enzyme. (1): D test, note flattering "D shape" zone of inhibition of clindamycin (CD) on the side of erythromycin (E) confirming production of erythromycin inducible methylase. (2): Note 18 mm zone of inhibition of cefoxitin disc, detection of MRSA.**

Methicillin resistant *Staphylococcus aureus* (MRSA)

In *S. aureus* cell wall formation involves transglycosylation (formation of linear monomers of sugar) and transpeptidation (interlinking of peptides to strengthen cell wall) processes. Binding of beta-lactam antibiotics on transpeptidation domain inhibit interlinking of peptides therefore a formation of weak cell wall which is easy to rapture and releasing of cytoplasmic contents hence cell death.

Methicillin resistant *S. aureus* (MRSA) is any *S. aureus* with ability to hydrolyze beta-lactam antibiotics; penicillins, cephalosporins and monobactam making the antibiotics ineffective. Resistance among *S. aureus* is encoded by chromosomal gene, *mec*A which is carried within staphylococcal chromosomal cassette "SCC" *mec*, a mobile genetic element. SCC may be horizontally transferred between *Staphylococcus* species, however, recently have been reported among *Streptococcus pneumoniae*. SCC is recombined into host bacteria genome and inserted near origin of replication by using two recombinase genes; *ccr*A and *ccr*B which are also contained within it. The mecA gene in MRSA is responsible for production of "penicillin binding protein 2A" (PBP2A) reducing beta-lactam antibiotics affinity towards bacterial cell wall [107-109].

174

When setting for antibiotic susceptibility testing, 30µg cefoxitin disc should be seeded together with other antibiotics discs which will be used as surrogate test for oxacillin sensitivity and phenotypically detects MRSA. *S. aureus* with zone of inhibition of equal or less than 21 mm should be reported as MRSA positive.

Extended spectrum beta-lactamase (ESBL) producing Enterobacteriaceae

Phenotypically, 30µg ceftazidime, 30µg ceftriaxone and 30µg cefpodoxime discs may be used to predict production of beta-lactamase enzymes from bacteria [110]. It is recommended that, all isolates of *Escherichia coli* and *Klebsiella* species isolated from in-patients should be tested for production of beta-lactamase enzymes simultaneously during performing antibiotics susceptibility testing [110]. For detection of SHV and TEM-ESBL producing bacteria, ceftazidime is the best while for detection of CTX-M-ESBL producing bacteria, ceftriaxone is the best [110]. Single antibiotic disc of cefpodoxime may be used alternatively to indicate presence of all ESBL families i.e SHV, TEM and CTX-M [110].

CLSI recommends the use of 30µg cefotaxime and 30µg ceftazidime, alone and in combination with clavulanic acid a beta-lactamase inhibitor to detect ESBL production among *Klebsiella pneumoniae*, *Klebsiella oxytoca*, *Escherichia coli* and *Proteus mirabillis* [105]. Clavulanic acid and cephalosporin antibiotics (cefotaxime or ceftazidime) acts synergistically. Clavulanic acid inhibits production of beta-lactamase enzymes making bacteria susceptible towards cephalosporin antibiotics. Any isolate with a difference of ≥ 5 mm in zone of diameters between cephalosporin antibiotics in combination with clavulanic acid and alone is confirmed ESBL producer.

Double disc synergy, a disk diffusion technique using 30µg amoxycillin-clavulanic acid, 30µg ceftriaxone and 30µg ceftazidime may be employed to detect ESBL production [111-113]. Briefly, ceftriaxone and ceftazidime discs are seeded edge by edge on sides of amoxycillin-clavulanic acid about 10-15 mm. Diffusion of clavulanic acid from amoxycillin-clavulanic acid disc will inhibit production of beta-lactamase enzymes making bacteria around this disc susceptible towards ceftriaxone and ceftazidime. Zones of inhibition of ceftriaxone and ceftazidime will be enhanced towards amoxycillin-clavulanic acid for positive ESBL producers [111, 112].

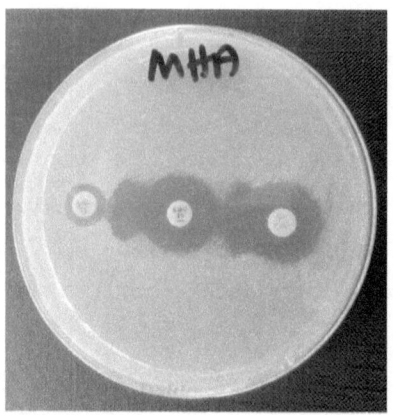

Figure 30: Enhanced zones of inhibitions of ceftriaxone and ceftazidime towards amoxycillin-clavulanic acid, a phenotypic confirmation of ESBL production

Carbapenemase producing *Enterobacteriaceae* and *Pseudomonas aeruginosa*

CLSI recommends the use of ertapenem for phenotypic detection of carbapenemase producing Enterobacteriaceae and Pseudomonas aeruginosa [114]. Non-susceptibility of test bacteria to one or more agents of carbapenem indicates production of carbapenemase; however ertapenem is the best indicator. Mostly, isolates resistant to carbapenem agents are also resistant to one or more agents of cephalosporin third generations. However, the scenario is not always the same, sometime, carbapenemase producing bacteria are sensitive to cephalosporins [114].

Modified Hodge test (MHT) also known as clover-leaf test is cost-effective and easy phenotypic confirmatory test for detection of carbapenemase production among members of *Enterobacteriaceae* [115]. Fresh grown *Escherichia coli* (ATCC 25922) is suspended into sterile physiological saline equivalent to 0.5McFarland turbidity standard solution. A lawn of this suspension is made on Muller Hinton agar (MHA) plate and left for 15 minutes on bench to dry before test organism is streaked. A 10µg meropenem or imipenem is seeded at the center of MHA plate and then test organism is streaked from the edge of the disc to plate's periphery. Plates should be incubated at 37⁰C overnight. Inward curved zone of inhibition (clover-leaf shape) of susceptible bacteria (*E. coli* ATCC 26922) attaching streak of test bacteria confirm production of carbapenemase [115].

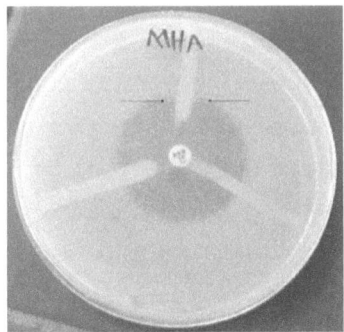

Figure 31: Modified Hodge test, phenotypic confirmation of carbapenemase production. Clover-leaf like appearance shown by arrows interpret positive production of carbapenemase enzyme

Immunodiagnostic techniques
Introduction

Antigen-antibody reaction is the key principle of detection (or diagnosis) of infection (or disease) of interest in immunodiagnostic assays. Back to 1960s when immunology was introduced as diagnostic tool to date, its technology is expanding and diversely applied because of its simplicity, liability (acceptable high sensitivity and specificity), and rapidity and cost effective. Antibody (or antigen) is conjugated with color forming enzyme or radio-label or fluorescent-label, as a probe it will react and detect antigen (or antibody) of interest. Applications of immunodiagnostic assays include Immunochromatography assays, latex agglutination assays and enzyme linked immune-sorbent assays (ELISAs).

Immunochromatography assay (ICA)

Immunochromatography assay (ICA) also known as lateral flow assay (LFA) is a capillary paper based strip intended to detect the presence (positive result) or absence (negative result) of targeted analyte in a complex mixture of analytes [116]. The materials of capillary paper on this test strip may be made from porous paper, microstructured polymer or sintered polymer which has the capacity to transport fluid spontaneously. Immunochromatography is a combination of immunochemical reactions to form antigen-antibody complex and chromatography a production of colored product (analyte) which was separated from a mixture of analytes. A specific biomolecule against antigen or antibody of interest is mobilized in a capillary paper along with some dyes to produces coloured lines [117]. ICA is a simple and yet cost effective device which does not need any specialization therefore it can be performed at home, point-of-care or in a clinical laboratory. Serum, plasma, whole blood and urine are widely used biological samples however other body fluids may be used [116]. Also, solid or semi-solid biological samples such as stool may be used after being buffered into liquid forms. Different bacterial infections such as syphilis and salmonella infections can be detected by this assays. Furthermore, markers of bacterial infections like C-reactive protein may also be detected.

Four major compartments of ICA

ICA device has four compartments of which all compartments are mounted on backing card just to provide assembling platform of all the compartments [118].

i. Sample application pad; is place where sample should be applied so as it can be transported to other compartments in a smooth, continuous and homogenous flow. The amount of sample to be applied and any pretreatment basically depends on manufacturer's instructions.

ii. Conjugate pad; at this compartment a labeled conjugate biomolecule (usually nano-colloid gold particle) is placed and upon contact with moving liquid sample it forms a complex with either antibody or antigen of interest.

iii. Substrate membrane; at this compartment test (T) and control (C) lines are drawn. Furthermore, at "T" line, antigens or antibodies intended to react with target analyte are immobilized to give either a positive or negative result and at "C" line ant-human antibodies are immobilized to give a positive control of device's procedure independent of test result.

iv. Adsorbent pad; this compartment at the end of test strip functions as a sink to absorb any excess fluid and to hold that fluid so as it may prevent back-flowing.

Principle of ICA

Liquid sample with or without analyte is applied to the sample application pad which subsequently flow to other compartments under capillary action. From sample application pad, the next compartment is conjugate pad. Flow may be facilitated by addition of buffered water or saline provided with test kit. At the conjugate pad, immobilized labeled antibodies capture target antigens and form labeled antibody-antigen complex or vice versa. This complex moves towards T line where it is captured by another antibodies fixed at this line forming labeled antibody-antigen (analyte)-primary antibody (fixed at T line) complex. Excess labeled antibodies flowing towards C line are captured by ant-human antibodies fixed at this line forming labeled antibody-anti-human antibody complex. Excess liquid sample or buffered liquid sample is absorbed by absorbing pad at adsorbent pad compartment. Primary antibody at T line captures analyte which is also captured by labeled-antibody at conjugate pad compartment. Therefore if no analyte captured, primary antibodies fixed at T line will not bind labeled antibodies and these labeled antibodies will flow to be captured by ant-human antibodies fixed at C line. Henceforth, presence of colored line at T line depends on the presence of target analyte in a sample while C line we always produce a colored line independent of the presence or absence of an analyte of target in a sample. Appearance of colored line at C line ensures the validity of a test strip [118].

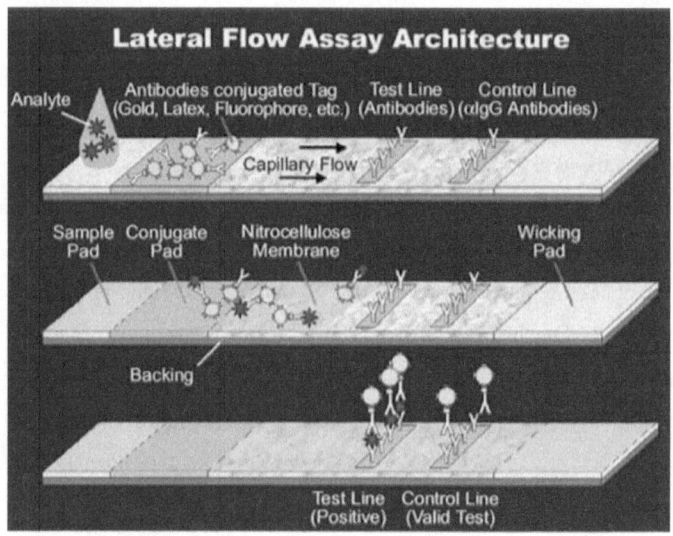

Figure 32: Illustration and principle of ICA (Source: U.S-NASA)

Interpretation of ICA results

Usually results are read within 5-30 minutes. Test is "POSITIVE" when both lines, T and C appears regardless of the intensity of color at T line. Test is "NEGATIVE" when only colored line appears at C line. Test is "INVALID" when no colored line at C line regardless of the presence or absence of line at T line.

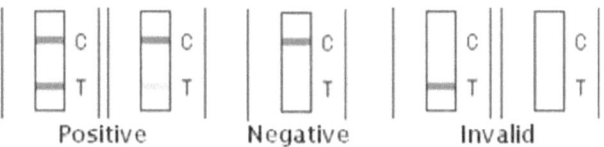

Positive   Negative   Invalid

Figure 33: Interpretations of ICA showing strong positive, weak positive, negative and invalid results from left to right (Source: Alibaba.com [119])

Latex agglutination assay

Latex agglutination reaction is observed when a sample containing specific antibody (or antigen) forms a visible clumping when mixed with an antigen (or antibody) coated on the surface of latex particles [120]. There are two types of latex agglutination test, active and passive. Active latex agglutination assay utilizes natural occurring antigens, for example; Brucella latex agglutination test for detection of brucellosis and Widal test for detection of typhoid fever by Salmonella typhi. Passive latex agglutination assay utilizes synthetic antigens when pathogenic culture is not feasible, for example; VDRL test for detection of syphilis. Other latex agglutination assay include *Clostridium difficile* toxins A and B, *Escherichia coli* 0157:H7 from culture colonies of *E coli*, anti-CRP antibodies for detection of C-reactive protein, detection of capsular antigens of *Hemophillus influenzae*, Meningococcus and Pneumococcus. Also, detection of *Cryptococcus neoformans* in cerebrospinal fluid for diagnosis of Cryptococcal meningitis [121]. Moreover, latex agglutination assay can be qualitative or quantitative. Qualitative latex agglutination assay observes the presence or absence of agglutination only. Quantitative latex agglutination assay is when serially diluted sample is reacted with the reagent and the maximum dilution reacted is the antibody (or antigen) titer.

Principle of latex agglutination assay

Antibodies are known to have two antigen binding sites therefore they can binds two antigens at a time. Polyvalent antigen allows binding of two or more antibodies on a single antigen. This kind of reaction between antibodies and polyvalent antigens result into a cross-linking between antibodies and antigens. If one between the two, antibodies or polyvalent antigens are coated on the surfaces of latex particles, visible clumping known as agglutination occurs [122]. Sometimes due to high antibody (or antigen) titer in client's sample, false negative result may happen. High titers interfere formation of particulate antibody (or antigen)-antigen (or antibody) complexes. This phenomenon is known as Prozone effect or Hook phenomenon [122].

Interpretation of latex agglutination assay

Sample preparation, procedures and exactly time to read and interpret results varies widely with test type and manufacturer. Generally, presence of visible agglutination is interpreted as "POSITIVE" and absence of visible agglutination is interpreted as "NEGATIVE".

Enzymes linked immune-sorbent assay (ELISA)

Introduction

ELISA is dated back to 1971 when it was introduced by Peter Perlmann and Eva Engvall at Stockholm University in Sweden. Simply, ELISA is the reaction between antigen and antibody to form colored complexes. The intensity of colored product depends on the concentration of detected analyte of target, antibody or antigen. Enzyme conjugated antibody (or antigen) is reacted with colorless chromogenic substrate to form a colored product [123]. Alkaline phosphatase (AP), beta galactosidase (BG) and horse radish peroxidase (HRP) are widely used enzymes. Also, ortho-phenyldiamine dihydrochloride (for horse radish peroxidase), chlorophenolred-beta-D-galactopyranoside (for beta galactosidase) and paranitrophenyl phosphate (for alkaline phosphatase) are some of common and specific substrates utilized [124]. All of these reactions of ELISA are taking place in 96 wells polystyrene plate [123].

Principles of ELISA

Principally there are four types of ELISA namely direct ELISA, indirect ELISA, sandwich ELISA and competitive ELISA. ELISA are categorized on the basis of series of reactions and patterns of antigen-antibody complexes formed. Therefore, principles of ELISA is hereby explained under each specific type. In any run, positive and negative control sera or any other applicable sample should be incorporated in an ELISA plate. Duration and conditions of incubation and type of color of final product varies widely depending on manufacturer.

Direct ELISA

This type of ELISA detects antigen. Microtiter well is coated with testing antigen (sample), sealed and incubated at 4^0C for overnight. Microtiter well is washed with 0.05% of Tween-20 in phosphate buffered saline (PBS-T). Bovine serum albumin (i.e 0.5g of milk in 50 ml of PBS) is used for blocking other binding sites. Microtiter well is then washed 3 times by using PBS-T to remove residues of bovine serum albumin. Horseradish peroxidase (HRP) conjugated to specific antibody (IgG) to coated antigen is added and incubated to allow a reaction resulting to antigen-antibody complexes. Microtiter plate (well) is washed 4-8 times using PBS-T to remove any unbound enzyme conjugated antibody. Then, substrate is added and incubated for 15-30 minutes to produce a visible colored product which is proportional to the concentration of antigen in a sample. Following addition of stop enzyme, $2N.H_2SO_4$, the reaction is stopped. Plate is read by using ELISA plate reader at 450n within 30 minutes [125-127].

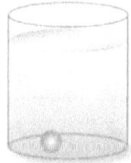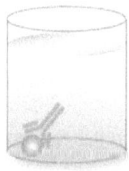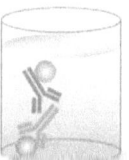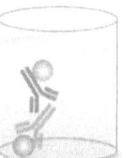

Figure 34: Illustrations of direct ELISA (Source: Bio-Rad [127])

Indirect ELISA

This type of ELISA detects antibody, specific antigen is coated on microtiter wells. Serum or any other applicable sample is added into microtiter wells to detect antibody of interest known as primary antibody. After specified of reaction to form antigen-antibody complexes, excess free primary antibodies and any other proteins are removed from microtiter wells by washing. Reagent containing enzyme conjugated antibodies known as secondary antibody is added and allowed to bind to primary antibody from serum (or sample) to form antigen-primary antibody-secondary antibody complexes. Unbound secondary antibodies are then removed by washing procedure. Specific substrate to enzyme conjugated on secondary antibody is added and allowed to react to produce a visible colored product. The intensity of color which is measured by spectrophotometer on ELISA plate reader is directly proportion to the concentration of antibodies of interest in a sample [123].

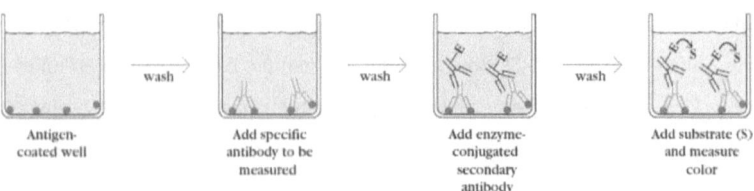

Antigen-coated well   Add specific antibody to be measured   Add enzyme-conjugated secondary antibody   Add substrate (S) and measure color

Figure 35: Illustrations of indirect ELISA (Source: Laboratory-Info [128])

Sandwich ELISA

This type of ELISA detect antigen, specific antibody is coated on microtiter wells. Sample containing antigen of interest is added and allowed to react with coated antibody (primary antibody) to form primary antibody-antigen complexes. Unbound antigens and other proteins are removed by washing. Secondary antibody conjugated to an enzyme is added and reacts with antigen bound to primary antibody on microtiter well to form primary antibody-antigen (sandwiched)-secondary enzyme linked antibody complexes. Excess unbound secondary enzyme linked antibodies are washed. Then, specific substrate to enzyme linked on secondary antibody is added for hydrolysis to produce a colored product. Again, the intensity of color is proportional to the concentration of antigen is a sample. Measuring of color intensity is done by spectrophotometer by using ELISA plate reader [123].

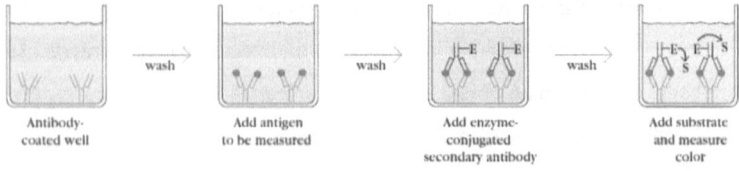

Antibody-coated well   Add antigen to be measured   Add enzyme-conjugated secondary antibody   Add substrate and measure color

Figure 36: Illustrations of sandwich ELISA (Source: Laboratory-Info [128])

Competitive ELISA

The name competitive ELISA come from the reality that sample antigen and the alike antigen coated to the microtiter wells are competing for specific antibody called primary antibody. Therefore, competitive ELISA detects antigen from a sample [128].

Sample containing antigen of interest is first incubated with specific antibody, reacting to form sample antigen-primary antibody complexes. This reaction is taking place outside the microtiter wells of ELISA. Then, this mixture containing sample antigen-primary antibody complexes is added into microtiter well were antigen similar to antigen of interest is coated. The more antigen in the sample, the more primary antibody will be bound during incubation therefore very few primary antibodies will be left unbound. Unbound primary antibody left will have to binds antigen coated on microtiter well, that very few primary antibody will bind and make microtiter well antigen-primary antibody complexes. Then secondary antibody linked to an enzyme is added to react with primary antibody bound on antigen coated on microtiter well to form antigen-primary antibody-secondary antibody complexes. Excess unbound secondary antibody are removed by washing followed by an addition of specific substrate. The substrate will hydrolyze enzyme on secondary antibody to produce a chromogenic product. The intensity of color is indirectly proportional the quantity of antigen present in a sample [128].

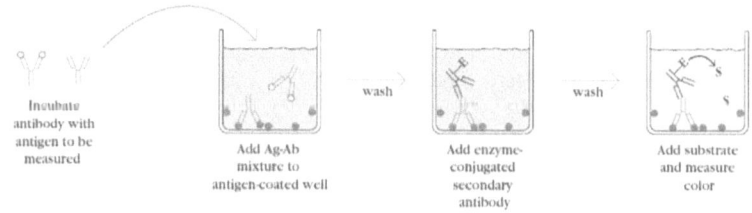

Incubate antibody with antigen to be measured

Add Ag-Ab mixture to antigen-coated well

wash

Add enzyme-conjugated secondary antibody

wash

Add substrate and measure color

Figure 37: Illustrations of competitive ELISA (Source: Laboratory-Info [128])

Interpretation of results from ELISA

Three different data output can be extracted from ELISA [128].

i. Qualitative: it's a POSITIVE (present) or NEGATIVE (absent) result of antibody (or antigen) of interest

ii. Semi-Quantitative: its relative comparison of antigen (or antibody) levels in samples.

iii. Quantitative: its relative comparison of antigen levels in samples with standard curve (a serial dilution of a known, purified antigen/antibody) in order to precisely calculate the quantity of antigen (or antibody) in various samples.

Advantage and disadvantage of each ELISA type of the other

Advantages and disadvantages of different types of ELISA [127]		
Type of ELISA	**Advantages**	**Disadvantages**
Direct	• Less prone to error – as less reagents and fewer steps are required	• Antigen immobilization is not specific - may cause higher background noise than indirect ELISA. Mainly because all proteins in the sample, including the target protein, will bind to the plate • Less flexible - each target protein needs a specific conjugated primary antibody • No signal amplification - reduces assay sensitivity
Indirect	• High sensitivity - more than one labeled secondary antibody can bind the primary antibody • Economical - fewer labeled antibodies are needed • Greater flexibility - different primary antibodies can be used with a single labeled secondary antibody	• Possibility of background noise - secondary antibody may be cross-reactive • Longer procedure than direct ELISA technique - additional incubation step for secondary antibody needed
Sandwich	• High sensitivity - 2-5 times more sensitive than direct or indirect ELISA • High specificity - two antibodies are involved in capture and detection • Flexibility - both direct and indirect detection can be used	• Antibody optimization can be difficult - cross-reactivity may occur between the capture and detection antibodies. Needs a standardized ELISA kit or tested antibody pair.

	• Best for: analysis of complex samples, since the antigen does not need to be purified prior to measurement.	
Competitive	• Main advantage - no sample processing is required and crude or impure samples can be used • More robust - less sensitive to sample dilution and sample matrix effects than the sandwich ELISA • More consistent - less variability between duplicate samples and assays • Maximum flexibility - it can be based on direct, indirect or sandwich ELISA • It is also suitable for detecting small antigens that cannot be bound by two different antibodies such as in the sandwich ELISA technique	

Safety in Bacteriology laboratory

Introduction

Laboratory safety means personal protection and protecting other laboratory members from infections due to infectious biological specimens and all accidents that may happen in the laboratory. Rules and guidelines are set to ensure safety is maintained in the laboratory all the time to every personnel.

Series of procedures in Bacteriology laboratory contains significant risks to laboratory staffs and clients. Such risks include but not limited to; exposure to infectious bacteria, exposure to corrosive and toxic chemicals, and physical injuries from laboratory accidents e.g burn accidents during operation of autoclave machine. To ensure safety in Bacteriology laboratory, personal protective gears should be worn all the time during procedures, laboratory safety rules and guidelines should be observed all the time, appropriate labeling of rooms, cabinets and reagents should be maintained. Laboratory customers or clients should be well instructed of possible dangers and how to keep safe. Any accident should be reported immediately for timely corrective and preventive action plans.

Laboratory safety rules and guidelines [129].

- Disinfect working benches every morning before working, after every complete procedure and during evening when leaving the laboratory. Disinfectant to use should be bactericidal, example 70% alcohol, 2% tincture of iodine.
- Always wear personal protective equipments (PPEs) when working on bench. Examples of PPEs are gloves, laboratory coats, goggles, masks and laboratory shoes.
- Always wash hands with soap and clean running tap water before and after laboratory procedures and after removing of gloves.
- In bacteriology laboratory, never take cultures outside laboratory room unless for critical purpose and biohazard packaging should be observed.
- Long hairs should be tied at the back to prevent contamination by touching on working benches surfaces.
- No open shoes like sandals are allowed in the laboratory.

- Highly infectious specimens should be processed in the biosafety cabinet. For example processing of sputum for tuberculosis infection should be done in biosafety cabinet level II.
- Never mouth pipette in the laboratory for any reason.
- Every biological specimen should be treated as highly infectious as it can be.
- Working bench should be neat and well organized; any unwanted material during performing procedures should be kept away.
- Any accident in the laboratory (spills, needle injury, and broken glasses) should be reported immediately so as immediate protective and preventive measures can be done.
- Dispose of waste materials appropriately in color coded waste disposal plastic bags. Sharp objects like needles and syringes should be kept in sharp boxes, anatomical infectious wastes like blood specimens should be kept in yellow colored waste bags, hard infectious wastes like dressings should be kept in red colored waste bags, infectious plastic wastes like syringes and gloves should be kept in blue colored waste bags and none infectious wastes like drinking water bottles should be kept in black colored waste bags.
- Disinfection and sterilization is a key role in bacteriology laboratory to ensure safety and prevention of infectious pathogens from patients' specimens to laboratory workers and the surrounding environment.

Disinfection and sterilization

Clinical bacteriology laboratory is an infectious area, because biological specimens from patients containing causative pathogens of infectious diseases are handled and through culture growth and multiplication of those pathogens is done. Routine adherence to personal protective gears, disinfection and sterilization of surfaces, equipments, supplies and culture plates with growth of bacteria should be well documented and implemented. In this chapter, sterilization will be discussed in detail.

Terminologies

Sterilization; is a process of complete killing or removal of all living microorganisms (bacteria, bacterial spores, fungi, protozoa and viruses) from surfaces or equipments [130].

Disinfection; is a process of destroying all harmful microorganisms from a surface or equipment by using disinfectant chemicals. Examples, 70% alcohol, Lysol, 2% iodine tincture, 10% povidone-iodine, 10% bleach (JIK) and 5% lysol [130].

Antiseptics; these are types of disinfectant which can be used on body surfaces to kill contaminating pathogens and reduce number of normal flora [131]. Examples: 70% alcohol, 2% iodine tincture and 10% povidone-iodine.

Asepsis; is a process of preventing microorganisms from reaching a protected surfaces or equipments. Example: manipulations in bacteriology laboratories such as during preparation of culture media.

Sterilization

Sterilization involves three major types, chemical, mechanical and physical sterilization techniques.

Physical sterilization; can be performed through; heat, radiation and filtration [130]. Heat sterilization can be dry heat or moist heat and it is reliable and can be performed in any setting. Dry heat sterilization can be accomplished by exposing material to be sterilized against naked flames. This method destroys oxidative processes of cells' components hence killing microorganisms [132]. For examples, incineration of infectious materials and equipments in an incinerator or direct heating of wire loops on spirits burner or Bunsen burner during culture process. Another method of dry heat sterilization is by using sterilizing oven at a temperature of 160 degree Celsius for 2 hours whereby killing of microorganisms is achieved by carbonization of their organic materials. Moist heat sterilization is achieved by using an autoclave machine, whereby rate of killing microorganisms' increases logarithmically with increasing temperature. The most important conditions to be maintained to ensure effective sterilization are temperature at 121 degree Celsius, pressure at 15 psi and time for 15 minutes after temperature and pressure has been reached [133, 134]. Pure saturated hot moist penetrate materials to be autoclaved hence killing all microorganisms including bacterial spores by completely destruction of proteinous parts of their cells. However, autoclaving can be limited by poor loading of materials for autoclaving, for example overcrowding of clothing materials may affect penetration of hot steam to the deep center of materials resulting to insufficient sterilization.

Chemical sterilization; this involves the use of chemical agents such as phenols (e.g. clearsol and stericol), chlorine releasing agents (e.g. sodium hypochlorite/jik/household bleach and calcium hypochlorite) and alcohols (70-95% alcohols). Effectiveness of chemical agent varies with type of microorganisms. Phenols are highly effective against viruses while chlorine releasing agents are highly effective against bacteria. Another limitation, chemicals are health hazardous, needs proper preventive measures, handling and disposal. Effectiveness of chemical agents disintegrates with storage and period conditions. Alcoholic chemical agents evaporate when they left open, hence lowering its effectiveness against microorganisms. Phenolic chemical agents lose its power when exposed to high temperature and light as its chlorine part is lost.

Mechanical sterilization: For sterilization of materials in solution forms whose chemical structures (active parts) should be maintained e.g. pharmaceutical solutions. Mechanical sterilization involves the use of membrane filtration technique. Materials are loaded on membrane filter, and then pressure is applied on top or vacuum is applied under the filter forcing materials to pass through small pores, 0.45 µm, of the filter. The pores size of the filter is smaller than microorganisms including viruses, hence trapping microorganisms on top of the membrane filter while keeping filtered solution sterile.

In bacteriology laboratory, potentially infectious materials such as inoculated culture plates with and without growth, used specimen containers and reusable wares (glass wares and autoclavable plastic wares) should be sterilized to avoid contamination and infection. Nature of materials to be sterilized in bacteriology laboratory and limitations of other types of sterilization methods limit to the use of physical sterilization by autoclave only.

Controls of physical sterilization

To ensure effective sterilization has achieved after autoclaving, controls should be incorporated during the process of sterilization. There are three types of sterilization control used in an autoclave; physical/mechanical, chemical and biological controls. Physical or mechanical sterilization control is by physical observation of temperature of 121 degree Celsius; pressure of 15 psi for 15 minutes has been reached through an *autoclave's gauge*. Chemical sterilization control is by using either *Browne's tubes* which contains solution that turns green from red after a temperature of 121 degree Celsius and pressure of 15 psi has reached, or *Bowie-Dick's tape* which contains cream diagonal lines which turns into blackish in the presence of high temperature and moist after complete sterilization (figure 1) [135]. Principle based to color change is a decomposition of lead carbonate to lead (II) oxide. Biological sterilization control is by using spore forming bacteria, the bacteria is incorporated in an autoclave as one among the materials to be sterilized. After complete process of sterilization, the bacteria are recovered by sub-culturing onto culture media. Growth of this control bacterium on culture medium means insufficient and ineffective sterilization and incapable of growth means sufficient and effective sterilization. Biological control bacteria used is *Bacillus stearothermophilus* [136].

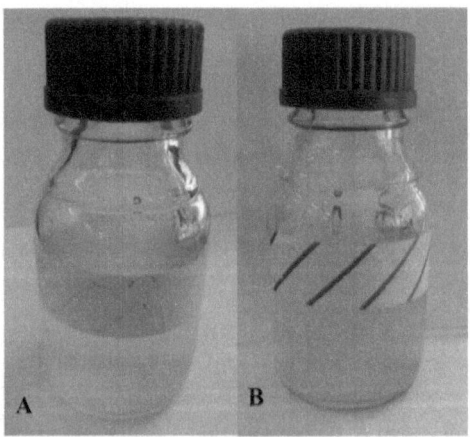

Figure 38; Sterilization control by Bowie-Dick's tape (A) before sterilization and (B) after sterilization by autoclaving

References

1. Popescu A, Doyle R: **The Gram stain after more than a century.** *Biotechnic & histochemistry* 1996, **71**(3):145-151.
2. Bartholomew JW, Mittwer T: **The gram stain.** *Bacteriological reviews* 1952, **16**(1):1.
3. Carbol-Fuchsin Z-N: **ACID-FAST BACTERIA-ZIEHL-NEELSEN STAIN (AFB).**
4. CDC: **Laboratory Evaluation Acid-Fast Bacilli Microbiology.** In.
5. Lucas S, Papadaki L, Conlon C, Sewankambo N, Goodgame R, Serwadda D: **Diagnosis of intestinal microsporidiosis in patients with AIDS.** *Journal of clinical pathology* 1989, **42**(8):885.
6. Cotte L, Rabodonirina M, Piens M, Perreard M, Mojon M, Trepo C: **Prevalence of intestinal protozoans in French patients infected with HIV.** *JAIDS Journal of Acquired Immune Deficiency Syndromes* 1993, **6**(9):1024-1029.
7. Henriksen SA, Pohlenz J: **Staining of cryptosporidia by a modified Ziehl-Neelsen technique.** *Acta Veterinaria Scandinavica* 1981, **22**(3-4):594-596.
8. Clarke S, McIntyre M: **Aci-fast bodies in faecal smears stained by the modified Ziehl-Neelsen technique.** *British journal of biomedical science* 2001, **58**(1):7.
9. Ridley D, Hawgood B: **The value of formol-ether concentration of faecal cysts and ova.** *Journal of Clinical Pathology* 1956, **9**(1):74.
10. **Lowenstein-Jensen (LJ) Medium- Composition, Principle, Uses, Preparation and Colony Morphology** [https://microbiologyinfo.com/lowenstein-jensen-lj-medium-composition-principle-uses-preparation-and-colony-morphology/]
11. **Löwenstein–Jensen (LJ) Medium: Prepartion and Uses** [https://microbeonline.com/preparation-uses-lowenstein-jensen-lj-medium/]
12. Hoberman A, Wald ER, Reynolds EA, Penchansky L, Charron M: **Pyuria and bacteriuria in urine specimens obtained by catheter from young children with fever.** *The Journal of pediatrics* 1994, **124**(4):513-519.
13. Thomas V, Shelokov A, Forland M: **Antibody-coated bacteria in the urine and the site of urinary-tract infection.** *New England Journal of Medicine* 1974, **290**(11):588-590.
14. Stamm WE, Norrby SR: **Urinary tract infections: disease panorama and challenges.** *The Journal of infectious diseases* 2001, **183**(Supplement_1):S1-S4.
15. Cheesbrough M: **District laboratory practice in tropical countries**: Cambridge university press; 2006.
16. Vandepitte J: **Basic laboratory procedures in clinical bacteriology**: World Health Organization; 2003.
17. Washington JA: **Urine culture contamination.** *Archives of pathology & laboratory medicine* 1998, **122**(2):120.
18. Schmiemann G, Kniehl E, Gebhardt K, Matejczyk MM, Hummers-Pradier E: **The diagnosis of urinary tract infection: a systematic review.** *Deutsches Ärzteblatt International* 2010, **107**(21):361.
19. Vaillancourt S, McGillivray D, Zhang X, Kramer MS: **To clean or not to clean: effect on contamination rates in midstream urine collections in toilet-trained children.** *Pediatrics* 2007, **119**(6):e1288-e1293.
20. Al-Orifi F, McGillivray D, Tange S, Kramer MS: **Urine culture from bag specimens in young children: are the risks too high?** *The Journal of pediatrics* 2000, **137**(2):221-226.

21.   Valenstein P, Meier F: **Urine culture contamination: a College of American Pathologists Q-Probes study of contaminated urine cultures in 906 institutions.** *Archives of pathology & laboratory medicine* 1998, **122**(2):123.
22.   Lauer B, Reller L, Mirrett S: **Evaluation of preservative fluid for urine collected for culture.** *Journal of clinical microbiology* 1979, **10**(1):42-45.
23.   Schumann GB, Greenberg NF: **Usefulness of macroscopic urinalysis as a screening procedure: a preliminary report.** *American journal of clinical pathology* 1979, **71**(4):452-456.
24.   Washington JA, White CM, Laganiere R, Michon, Smith LH: **Detection of significant bacteriuria by microscopic examination of urine.** *Laboratory Medicine* 2016, **12**(5):294-296.
25.   Sultana RV, Zalstein S, Cameron P, Campbell D: **Dipstick urinalysis and the accuracy of the clinical diagnosis of urinary tract infection.** *The Journal of emergency medicine* 2001, **20**(1):13-19.
26.   Simerville JA, Maxted WC, Pahira JJ: **Urinalysis: a comprehensive review.** *Am Fam Physician* 2005, **71**(6):1153-1162.
27.   Aspevall O, Osterman B, Dittmer R, Stén L, Lindbäck E, Forsum U: **Performance of four chromogenic urine culture media after one or two days of incubation compared with reference media.** *Journal of clinical microbiology* 2002, **40**(4):1500-1503.
28.   Weinstein MP: **Blood culture contamination: persisting problems and partial progress.** *Journal of clinical microbiology* 2003, **41**(6):2275-2278.
29.   Riedel S, Bourbeau P, Swartz B, Brecher S, Carroll KC, Stamper PD, Dunne WM, McCardle T, Walk N, Fiebelkorn K: **Timing of specimen collection for blood cultures from febrile patients with bacteremia.** *Journal of clinical microbiology* 2008, **46**(4):1381-1385.
30.   Schifman RB, Pindur A: **The effect of skin disinfection materials on reducing blood culture contamination.** *American journal of clinical pathology* 1993, **99**(5):536-538.
31.   Weinstein MP: **Current blood culture methods and systems: clinical concepts, technology, and interpretation of results.** *Clinical infectious diseases* 1996, **23**(1):40-46.
32.   Hoffman SL, Edman DC, Punjabi NH, Lesmana M, Cholid A, Sundah S, Harahap J: **Bone marrow aspirate culture superior to streptokinase clot culture and 8 ml 1: 10 blood-to-broth ratio blood culture for diagnosis of typhoid fever.** *The American Journal of Tropical Medicine and Hygiene* 1986, **35**(4):836-839.
33.   Washington JA, Ilstrup DM: **Blood cultures: issues and controversies.** *Reviews of infectious diseases* 1986, **8**(5):792-802.
34.   Surase P, Nataraj G, Pattamadai K, Mehta P, Pazare A, Agarwal M, Nanavati R: **An appropriately performed conventional blood culture can facilitate choice of therapy in resource-constrained settings-comparison with BACTEC 9050.** *Journal of postgraduate medicine* 2016, **62**(4):228.
35.   Center WFBM: **New BD BACTEC Blood   Culture System.** In.; 2015.
36.   Stotts NA, Whitney JD: **Identifying and evaluating wound infection.** *Home Healthcare Now* 1999, **17**(3):159-164.
37.   Bagnall NM, Vig S, Trivedi P: **Surgical-site infection.** *Surgery (Oxford)* 2009, **27**(10):426-430.
38.   Cutting KF: **Wound exudate: composition and functions.** *British journal of community nursing* 2003, **8**(Sup3):S4-S9.

39. Sharma M, Bhatia V: **Abdominal tuberculosis**. *Indian Journal of Medical Research* 2004, **120**(4):305.

40. Bonham PA: **Swab cultures for diagnosing wound infections: a literature review and clinical guideline**. *Journal of Wound Ostomy & Continence Nursing* 2009, **36**(4):389-395.

41. Tyagi A, Kapil A, Singh P: **Incidence of methicillin resistant Staphylococcus aureus (MRSA) in pus samples at a tertiary care hospital, AIIMS, New Delhi**. *J Indian Acad Clin Med* 2008, **9**(1):33-35.

42. Cox CD, Adams P: **Siderophore activity of pyoverdin for Pseudomonas aeruginosa**. *Infection and immunity* 1985, **48**(1):130-138.

43. Rissing JP, Crowder JG, Dunfee T, White A: **Bacteroides bacteremia from decubitus ulcers**. *Southern medical journal* 1974, **67**(10):1179-1182.

44. Winn WC: **Koneman's color atlas and textbook of diagnostic microbiology**: Lippincott williams & wilkins; 2006.

45. Wasfy M, Oyofo B, Elgindy A, Churilla A: **Comparison of preservation media for storage of stool samples**. *Journal of clinical microbiology* 1995, **33**(8):2176-2178.

46. Stokes J, Osborne W: **A selenite brilliant green medium for the isolation of Salmonella**. *Applied microbiology* 1955, **3**(4):217.

47. Lesmana M, Rockhill R, Sutanti D, Sutomo A: **An evaluation of alkaline peptone water for enrichment of Vibrio cholerae in feces**. *The Southeast Asian journal of tropical medicine and public health* 1985, **16**(2):265-267.

48. Gomez JR, Salinas IL, Salmerón JP, Cordoba ES, Campos LM: **Evaluation of methods for isolation of Salmonella species using modified semisolid Rappaport-Vassiliadis medium and Salmonella-Shigella agar**. *European Journal of Clinical Microbiology and Infectious Diseases* 1998, **17**(11):791-793.

49. Zige DV, Ohimain EI, Sridhar K: **Enteric Bacteria from ready to eat food vended in Amassoma community in Niger Delta and its health implication**. *IOSR Journal of Environmental Science, Toxicology And Food Technology (IOSR-JESTFT)* 2013, **6**(4):62-65.

50. Maddocks S, Olma T, Chen S: **Comparison of CHROMagar Salmonella medium and xylose-lysine-desoxycholate and Salmonella Shigella agars for isolation of Salmonella strains from stool samples**. *Journal of clinical microbiology* 2002, **40**(8):2999-3003.

51. **Thiosulfate Citrate bile salts sucrose (TCBS) agar: Composition, uses and colony characteristics** [https://microbeonline.com/thiosulfate-citrate-bile-salts-sucrose-tcbs-agarcomposition-uses-colony-characteristics/]

52. **TCBS (THIOSULFATE CITRATE BILE SALTS SUCROSE) AGAR** [https://catalog.hardydiagnostics.com/cp_prod/content/hugo/TCBSAgar.htm]

53. **CAMPYLOBACTER BLOOD-FREE SELECTIVE MEDIUM (MODIFIED CCDA- PRESTON)** [http://www.oxoid.com/UK/blue/prod_detail/prod_detail.asp?pr=SR0155&cat=&c=UK &lang=EN]

54. Greenwood D: **Medical Microbiology: A Guide to Microbial Infections: Pathogenesis, Immunity, Laboratory Diagnosis and Control. New York: Churchill Livingstone**. In.: Elsevier; 2012.

55. Church DL: **Cerebrospinal Fluid Cultures**. In. *Clinical Microbiology Procedures Handbook, Fourth Edition*. edn.: American Society of Microbiology; 2016: 3.7. 1 3.7. 11.

56. Thakur R, Goyal R, Sarma S: **Laboratory Diagnosis of Tuberculous Meningitis–Is There a Scope for Further Improvement?** *Journal of laboratory physicians* 2010, **2**(1):21.

57. Chen P, Shi M, Feng G-D, Liu J-Y, Wang B-J, Shi X-D, Ma L, Liu X-D, Yang Y-N, Dai W: **A highly efficient Ziehl-Neelsen stain: identifying de novo intracellular Mycobacterium tuberculosis and improving detection of extracellular M. tuberculosis in cerebrospinal fluid.** *Journal of clinical microbiology* 2012, **50**(4):1166-1170.

58. Greenlee J: **Approach to diagnosis of meningitis. Cerebrospinal fluid evaluation.** *Infectious disease clinics of North America* 1990, **4**(4):583-598.

59. Chuck SL, Sande MA: **Infections with Cryptococcus neoformans in the acquired immunodeficiency syndrome.** *New England Journal of Medicine* 1989, **321**(12):794-799.

60. Park BJ, Wannemuehler KA, Marston BJ, Govender N, Pappas PG, Chiller TM: **Estimation of the current global burden of cryptococcal meningitis among persons living with HIV/AIDS.** *Aids* 2009, **23**(4):525-530.

61. Heo EY, Shin S, Chung HS, Jeong Y-J, Oh SH, Kim DK: **The effect of using blood culture bottle of bronchoalveolar larvage fluid in pneumonia.** *BMC infectious diseases* 2016, **16**(1):247.

62. Yagupsky P, Peled N, Press J: **Use of BACTEC 9240 blood culture system for detection of Brucella melitensis in synovial fluid.** *Journal of clinical microbiology* 2001, **39**(2):738-739.

63. Jain N, Lodha R, Kabra S: **Upper respiratory tract infections.** *Indian journal of pediatrics* 2001, **68**(12):1135-1138.

64. Melio FR, Holmes D: **Upper respiratory tract infections.** *Emergency Medicine St Louis: Mosby* 1998:1529-1553.

65. Kidenya BR, Kabangila R, Peck RN, Mshana SE, Webster LE, Koenig SP, Johnson Jr WD, Fitzgerald DW: **Early and efficient detection of Mycobacterium tuberculosis in sputum by microscopic observation of broth cultures.** *PLoS One* 2013, **8**(2):e57527.

66. Seni J, Kidenya BR, Obassy E, Mirambo M, Burushi V, Mazigo HD, Kapesa A, Majigo M, Mshana SE: **Low sputum smear positive tuberculosis among pulmonary tuberculosis suspects in a tertiary hospital in Mwanza, Tanzania.** *Tanzania journal of health research* 2012, **14**(2).

67. Chang AB, Chang CC, O'Grady K, Torzillo P: **Lower respiratory tract infections.** *Pediatric Clinics of North America* 2009, **56**(6):1303-1321.

68. Finegold SM, Johnson CC: **Lower respiratory tract infection.** *The American journal of medicine* 1985, **79**(5):73-77.

69. Jawetz EM, Adelberg I: **Review of medical microbiology.** 1980.

70. Johnson AL, Hampson DF, Hampson NB: **Sputum color: potential implications for clinical practice.** *Respiratory care* 2008, **53**(4):450-454.

71. Karnath B, Agyeman A, Lai A: **Pneumococcal pneumonia: update on therapy in the era of antibiotic resistance.** *Consultant* 2003, **43**(3):321-327.

72. Ledbetter EO: **Pneumococcal pneumonia in children.** *Patient Care* 1989, **23**(9):117-129.

73. Gordon-Smith T: **Structure and function of red and white blood cells.** *Medicine* 2009, **37**(3):119-124.

74. Small P, Gaskins D, Rand K, Huang S-W: **Diagnostic system for differentiating sputum from saliva.** In.: Google Patents; 2002.

75. Fritz JM, McDonald JR: **Osteomyelitis: approach to diagnosis and treatment.** *The Physician and sportsmedicine* 2008, **36**(1):50-54.

76. Jacob E, Durham L, Falk M, Williams T, Wheat L: **Antibody response to teichoic acid and peptidoglycan in Staphylococcus aureus osteomyelitis**. *Journal of clinical microbiology* 1987, **25**(1):122-127.

77. Senneville E, Melliez H, Beltrand E, Legout L, Valette M, Cazaubie M, Cordonnier M, Caillaux M, Yazdanpanah Y, Mouton Y: **Culture of percutaneous bone biopsy specimens for diagnosis of diabetic foot osteomyelitis: concordance with ulcer swab cultures**. *Clinical infectious diseases* 2006, **42**(1):57-62.

78. Mijuskovic B, Kuehl R, Widmer A, Jundt G, Frei R, Gürke L, Wolff T: **Culture of bone biopsy specimens overestimates rate of residual osteomyelitis after toe or forefoot amputation**. *The Journal of bone and joint surgery American volume* 2018, **100**(17):1448.

79. Elmer W, Stephen DA, William M, Paul C, Washington C: **Color atlas and textbook of diagnostic microbiology**. In.: Philadelphia: Lippincott; 1992.

80. Stuart C, Van Stratum E, Rustigian R: **Further studies on urease production by Proteus and related organisms**. *Journal of bacteriology* 1945, **49**(5):437.

81. Biomerieux: **Identification system for Enterobacteriaceae and other non-fastidious Gram-negative rods**. In.; 2002.

82. Tenover FC: **Antimicrobial Susceptibility Testing Methods for Bacterial Pathogens**. *Antimicrobial Drug Resistance* 2009:1151-1159.

83. Jorgensen JH, Ferraro MJ: **Antimicrobial susceptibility testing: general principles and contemporary practices**. *Clinical Infectious Diseases* 1998:973-980.

84. Lalitha M: **Manual on antimicrobial susceptibility testing**. *Performance standards for antimicrobial testing: Twelfth Informational Supplement* 2004, **56238**:454-456.

85. Au WY: **Broad-spectrum antibiotics**. *The American journal of nursing* 1964:105-109.

86. Saene R, Fairclough S, Petros A: **Broad-and narrow-spectrum antibiotics: a different approach**. *Clinical Microbiology and Infection* 1998, **4**(1):56-57.

87. Acar J: **Broad-and narrow-spectrum antibiotics: An unhelpful categorization**. *Clinical Microbiology and Infection* 1997, **3**(4):395-396.

88. Wiegand I, Hilpert K, Hancock RE: **Agar and broth dilution methods to determine the minimal inhibitory concentration (MIC) of antimicrobial substances**. *Nature protocols* 2008, **3**(2):163.

89. Andrews JM: **Determination of minimum inhibitory concentrations**. *Journal of antimicrobial Chemotherapy* 2001, **48**(suppl 1):5-16.

90. Sandle T: **Pharmaceutical microbiology: essentials for quality assurance and quality control**: Woodhead Publishing; 2015.

91. Nachnani S, Scuteri A, Newman MG, Avanessian AB, Lomeli SL: **E-test: A new technique for antimicrobial susceptibility testing for periodontal microorganisms**. *Journal of periodontology* 1992, **63**(7):576-583.

92. Acharya T: **E-TEST (Epsilometer test): Principle, purpose, procedure, results and interpretations**. In.; 2015.

93. Biomerieux: **VITEK 2**. In.

94. Badawy AS: **Detection of Genes Encoding for Metallo-β-lactamases produced by Resistant Acinetobacter baumannii and Pseudomonas spp. isolated from Clinical Specimens in Ramadi**. Ministry of Higher Education; 2013.

95. Pincus DH: **Microbial identification using the bioMérieux Vitek® 2 system**. *Encyclopedia of Rapid Microbiological Methods Bethesda, MD: Parenteral Drug Association* 2006.

96. Laboratories GHS: **Vitek 2 Compact – Identification and Susceptibility Testing**. In.; 2018.

97. Ligozzi M, Bernini C, Bonora MG, de Fatima M, Zuliani J, Fontana R: **Evaluation of the VITEK 2 system for identification and antimicrobial susceptibility testing of medically relevant gram-positive cocci**. *Journal of clinical microbiology* 2002, **40**(5):1681-1686.

98. Diagnostics FfIN: **MGIT Procedure Manual**. In.; 2006.

99. WHO: **Mycobacteriology Laboratory Manual: global laboratory initiative advancing TB diagnosis**. In.; 2014.

100. Heifets L, Linder T, Sanchez T, Spencer D, Brennan J: **Two liquid medium systems, mycobacteria growth indicator tube and MB redox tube, for Mycobacterium tuberculosis isolation from sputum specimens**. *Journal of clinical microbiology* 2000, **38**(3):1227-1230.

101. **Lowenstein-Jensen (LJ) Medium- Composition, Principle, Uses, Preparation and Colony Morphology** [https://microbiologyinfo.com/lowenstein-jensen-lj-medium-composition-principle-uses-preparation-and-colony-morphology/]

102. WHO: **Xpert MTB/RIF implementation manual: Technical and operational 'how-to': practical considerations**. In.; 2014.

103. **GeneXpert MTB/RIF Assay: Principle, Procedure, Results and Interpretations** [https://microbeonline.com/genexpert-mtbrif-assay-principle-procedure-results-interpretations/]

104. Shinnick TM, Starks AM, Alexander HL, Castro KG: **Evaluation of the Cepheid Xpert MTB/RIF assay**. *Expert review of molecular diagnostics* 2015, **15**(1):9-22.

105. Patel JB: **Performance standards for antimicrobial susceptibility testing**: Clinical and Laboratory Standards Institute; 2017.

106. Gadepalli R, Dhawan B, Mohanty S, Kapil A: **Inducible clindamycin resistance in clinical isolates of Staphylococcus aureus**. *Indian Journal of Medical Research* 2006, **123**(4):571.

107. Wang L, Archer GL: **Roles of CcrA and CcrB in excision and integration of staphylococcal cassette chromosome mec, a Staphylococcus aureus genomic island**. *Journal of bacteriology* 2010, **192**(12):3204-3212.

108. Lowy FD: **Antimicrobial resistance: the example of Staphylococcus aureus**. *The Journal of clinical investigation* 2003, **111**(9):1265-1273.

109. Ito T, Kuwahara-Arai K, Katayama Y, Uehara Y, Han X, Kondo Y, Hiramatsu K: **Staphylococcal cassette chromosome mec (SCCmec) analysis of MRSA**. In: *Methicillin-Resistant Staphylococcus Aureus (MRSA) Protocols*. edn.: Springer; 2014: 131-148.

110. Andrews J: **Detection of extended-spectrum b-lactamases (ESBLs) in E. coli and Klebsiella species**. In.; 2012.

111. Ahmed OI, El-Hady SA, Ahmed TM, Ahmed IZ: **Detection of bla SHV and bla CTX-M genes in ESBL producing Klebsiella pneumoniae isolated from Egyptian patients with suspected nosocomial infections**. *Egyptian Journal of Medical Human Genetics* 2013, **14**(3):277–283.

112. CLSI C: **Performance of standards for antimicrobial disk susceptibility tests; approved standards**. In.: Clinical and Laboratory Standard Institute Wayne, PA. USA; 2009.

113. Jarlier V, Nicolas M-H, Fournier G, Philippon A: **Extended broad-spectrum β-lactamases conferring transferable resistance to newer β-lactam agents in Enterobacteriaceae: hospital prevalence and susceptibility patterns**. *Clinical Infectious Diseases* 1988, **10**(4):867-878.

114. Wyne P: **Performance Standards for Antimicrobial Susceptibility Testing.** . In., 28th ed edn: Clinical and Laboratory Standards Institute; 2018.
115. Ramana K, Ratna Rao C, Kareem M, Reddy LR, Mani MR: **Modified Hodge test: a useful and the low-cost phenotypic method for detection of carbapenemase producers in Enterobacteriaceae members.** *Journal of natural science, biology, and medicine* 2013, **4**(2):346.
116. Koczula KM, Gallotta A: **Lateral flow assays.** *Essays in biochemistry* 2016, **60**(1):111-120.
117. Sebastian C, William H: **Immunochromatography: Formats and Applications.** *Indo American Journal of Pharmaceutical Research [Internett]* 2016, **6**(07).
118. **Immunochromatography Guide** [https://www.creative-diagnostics.com/Immunochromatography-guide.htm]
119. **High tech Salmonella rapid test food** [https://www.alibaba.com/product-detail/high-tech-Salmonella-Rapid-test-Food_60380025023.html]
120. Audrey Wanger VC, Richard S.P. Huang, Amer Wahed, Jeffrey K. Actor, Amitava Dasgupta: **Microbiology and Molecular Diagnosis in Pathology:** ELSEVIER; 2017.
121. **Latex Agglutination Test** [https://microbenotes.com/latex-agglutination-test/]
122. **Latex Agglutination** [https://vlab.amrita.edu/?sub=3&brch=69&sim=195&cnt=1]
123. **ELISA- Principle, Types and Applications** [http://microbiologynotes.com/elisa-principle-types-and-applications/]
124. Aydin S: **A short history, principles, and types of ELISA, and our laboratory experience with peptide/protein analyses using ELISA.** *Peptides* 2015, **72**:4-15.
125. **Direct ELISA** [https://www.sinobiological.com/direct-elisa.html]
126. **ELISA Test Procedures** [https://www.biochain.com/general/elisa-test-procedures/]
127. **Types of ELISA** [https://www.bio-rad-antibodies.com/elisa-types-direct-indirect-sandwich-competition-elisa-formats.html#Direct]
128. **ELISA : Principle, Procedure, Types, Applications and Animation** [https://laboratoryinfo.com/elisa/]
129. Kaufman JA: **Laboratory safety guidelines.** *AMERICAN LABORATORY* 1991, **23**(9):52-52.
130. Rutala W, Weber D: **Infection control: the role of disinfection and sterilization.** *Journal of Hospital Infection* 1999, **43**:S43-S55.
131. Patterson AM: **Meaning of "Antiseptic," "Disinfectant" and Related Words.** *American Journal of Public Health and the Nations Health* 1932, **22**(5):465-472.
132. Bruch C: **Some biological and physical factors in dry heat sterilization: a general review.** *Life sciences and space research* 1964, **2**:357-371.
133. **Combined autoclave and control system and method therefor.** In.: Google Patents; 1971.
134. Larsson RP, Witonsky RJ: **Temperature responsive sterility indicator.** In.: Google Patents; 1976.
135. Buglino ST, Patel PJ, Rahimzadeh BB: **Bowie-dick test device.** In.: Google Patents; 1993.
136. Hayakawa I, Kanno T, Yoshiyama K, Fujio Y: **Oscillatory compared with continuous high pressure sterilization on Bacillus stearothermophilus spores.** *Journal of Food Science* 1994, **59**(1):164-167.

CHAPTER FIVE

Healthcare associated infections (HCAIs)

HCAIs are those infections acquired by patients while receiving healthcare services in a time period of more than 48 hours in the hospital [1, 2]. Occasionally, healthcare workers (HCWs) may develop HCAIs [2]. Immunocompromised patients, patients colonized with antibiotic resistant bacteria, patients requiring intensive medical care and patients with multiple invasive procedures are at high risk of developing HCAIs [1, 2]. Basically, pathogenic microorganisms are transmitted by the following major routes; contact, airborne, droplets, vector-borne and common vehicles. Patients admitted in invasive care units (ICUs) develop HCAIs mostly catheter associated urinary tract infection (CA-UTI), central line associated bloodstream infection (CLABSI), ventilator associated pneumonia, surgical site infection (SSI), and *Clostridium difficile* (*C. diff*) infection. The burden of HCAIs is prevalent in low and middle income countries when compared to higher income countries [3]. In low and middle income countries, prevalence of HCAIs range from 5.7% to 19.1% with a pooled prevalence of 10.1% with most frequently reported HCAIs being SSI (29.1%) followed by UTIs (23.9%) and bloodstream infection (19.1%). In higher income countries the burden ranges from 3.5% to 12% with a pooled prevalence of 7.6%. Most frequently reported HCAIs was UTI (27-36%) followed by SSI (20%) [3]. In ICUs where antibiotic pressure and antimicrobial resistance (AMR) are high, patients develop HCAIs with AMR-bacteria. Consequently, the rate of morbidity and mortality is very high in these units [4, 5]. Every patient in ICU is supposed to be screened for any colonization with multidrug resistant (MDR) bacteria. Any colonized patient should be isolated (when necessary) and attended by special assigned HCWs with highly observation and adherence to protocols of infection prevention and control (IPC) to prevent possible cross-transmission to other patients and become the source of hospital outbreak [6]. Also, it is recommended that contact precautions are well observed to avoid acquisition of HCAIs and emerging of hospital outbreaks.

Therefore, the primary goal of any healthcare facility is to prevent HCAIs to patients, healthcare workers and all other visitors by focusing efforts to the major routes of infections transmission. Achieving this goal ensures minimum risk of occurrences of hospital outbreaks unless for emerging pathogens. Therefore, at all time, hospital management and authorities should observe adherence of HWCs to IPC domains. The domains include standard precautions, review and training of HCWs on IPCs and surveillance of MDR-bacteria.

Standard precautions

These are minimum practices of infection prevention that should be observed and adhered at all time during the care of all patients [7]. These basic precautions for infection prevention and control intend to protect patients and HCWs from HCAIs, but also prevent HCWs from transmitting of infectious pathogens between patients from recognized and unrecognized sources. This domain includes hand hygiene; safe injection practice (injection safety); availability of quality and proper use of personal protective equipment (PPEs); environmental cleaning and disinfection (safe and proper handling of patient contaminated immediate surfaces or equipment) and respiratory hygiene/cough etiquette.

Hand hygiene

This simple but most effective procedure is intended in prevention of cross-transmission of potentially infectious or pathogenic bacteria from one patient to another, from patient to HCW and from HCW to patient. The procedure takes about 1 minute but it is very important practice in prevention of HCAIs. Hand hygiene can be performed by washing hands with running water and liquid soap or antiseptic solutions, or by using hand sanitizers. Washing hands by using running water and antiseptic solution is performed prior to major invasive procedures such as surgery. But, sometimes hand sanitizers are not effective when hands are visibly soiled (or dirty), after taking care of known or suspected diarrheagenic patient with viral infection such as Norovirus or *C. diff* [7].

World Health Organization (WHO) in 2009 introduced the "five moments for hand hygiene" for the aim of reducing the burden of HCAIs [8, 9]. Those moments are 1. Before patient contact to protect the patient from pathogenic microorganism of HCW's hands; 2. Before aseptic procedure to protect the patient from pathogenic microorganism including patient's own germs from entering him/her; 3. After exposure to body fluid; 4. After patient contact and 5. After contact with patient immediate environment. The last three moments (3-4) aims to protect HCW from infection and hospital environment from contamination with harmful microorganism [9].

Personal protective equipments (PPEs)

Personal protective equipments include but not limited to gloves of all types, gowns, googles, aprons, gum boats and respirator masks. PPEs create barrier between patient and HCW therefore protecting HCW from acquiring contamination or infection from patient. Before putting on PPEs, HCW is supposed to assess the risk of exposure for proper and appropriate selection and wearing of PPEs. It is the legal task of employer to provide PPEs of acceptable quality, fit (to all HCWs) and available at every point of use. Also, provide training on proper use and disposal of PPEs. It should be mandatory that, HCWs attend IPC training on proper use and disposal PPEs and attendance records kept available [10].

Environmental cleaning and disinfection

Routine general cleanliness is emphasized at all places of healthcare facility following adequate protocols locally and internationally adopted and accepted. Documents of the protocols should put available in each ward or unit or clinic. For the aim of removing dirty and decontamination, cleaning by clean water and detergent is recommended. However in some circumstances such as during hospital outbreak, surfaces and equipments should be disinfected [10, 11].

Disinfection is the removal of potentially pathogenic bacteria to a minimum level which poses no risk of infections to patients or other people. Before disinfection, surfaces and equipments should be cleaned by clean water and detergent. Best disinfectant is chlorine releasing agents or chlorine dioxide solution because they are effective of killing both bacteria and viruses. When applied on metallic equipment, they should be rinsed off with clean water because hypochlorite is corrosive on these surfaces [10].

Types of cleaning are routine general cleaning, enhanced cleaning and terminal cleaning. *Routine general cleaning* is done at least once in daily basis however if surfaces or equipments are visibly soiled they should be disinfected after thorough leaning [10]. *Enhanced cleaning* is done at least twice in daily basis especially on frequently contacted surfaces or equipments during hospital outbreak or increased incidence of certain pathogenic bacteria. However sometimes more frequently cleaning in a day may be required for example cleaning of sanitary areas during diarrhea outbreaks [10]. **Terminal cleaning** is thorough cleaning or disinfection during outbreak or increased incidence of certain pathogenic bacteria, after patient discharge or transfer and after patient death [10].

Injection safety (safe injection practices)

Refers to proper and safer use (or handling) of all sharp objects (e.g., needles, intra-venous lines, syringes, medication vials e.t.c) during medical procedures to prevent blood-borne infections to patients, HCWs and others. Improper practices of injections during routine procedures in the hospital have resulted into 50 outbreaks of blood-borne viral infections including Hepatitis B and C viruses (HBV and HCV) [12]. These outbreaks are the result of negligence of following safe injection practices and aseptic techniques such as contamination of multi-dose vials with unclean syringes, re-using of syringes, re-using end-caps from single-use syringes, using single-dose vials for multiple patients, using uncleaned finger-stick devices on multiple patients and using of uncleaned blood sugar measuring devices on multiple patients [12].

Safe waste management

Safe management of healthcare waste reduces the potential risk to patients, HCWs, environment and general public. Waste produced in the course of healthcare procedures pose hazardous risk because they harbor potentially infectious microorganisms, contaminated needles, radioactive materials, genotoxic and hazardous chemical or pharmaceuticals. Improper waste separation, handling and disposal contaminates environment (soil, water and air) making it a potential source of infection epidemics. For example, about 21 million cases of HBV infections accounting to 32% of new cases, 2 million cases of HCV accounting to 40% of new cases and 260,000 cases of human immunodeficiency virus (HIV) infections accounting to 5% of new cases are due to improper injection practices and disposal [13, 14].

Healthcare wastes are categorized into two major classes: hazardous and non-hazardous wastes. Non-hazardous waste (e.g., empty water bottles, food remnant, and paper towels used for drying hands) does not pose any infection or injury risks and they are generally similar to household wastes. Hazardous wastes pose infection and/or injury risks because they are naturally infectious and potential in causing injury [13].

Review and training of HCWs on IPCs

IPC committee is comprised with a wide representation of stakeholders around the facility, including administrators, heads of clinical departments, physicians, nurses, and support services staff [15]. Support services staff include central supply, clinical microbiology laboratory, maintenance, pharmacy, housekeeping, orderlies, environmental services, training, waste management, and others [15]. Key hospital staffs form and maintain an active IPC committee which is comprised with representatives from different wards and units, including laboratory (bacteriology/microbiology), procurement, and sterilization and environmental cleaning. In small facilities (e.g., dispensaries), committee may consist of only two or three individuals because most of these functions overlap. It is the purpose of this committee to guide and support effective use of recommended IPC practices [15]. Also, this committee participates in reviewing, developing, and approving the facility's IPC policies as well as the yearly risk assessment, goals, and program evaluation. Any related problems that may arise after the review is resolved appropriately. Furthermore, in regular basis the IPC committee should review the status of HAIs at the facility and the effectiveness of IPC measures designed to combat them [15].

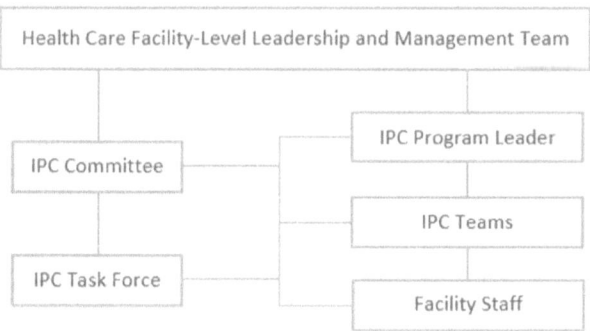

Figure 1: Organogram of IPC committee (Source: Infection Prevention and Control Program Management, Jhpiego Corporation, 2018)

The key responsibilities (activities) of the IPC team (adopted from: Infection Prevention and Control Program Management, Jhpiego Corporation, 2018 [15]) are:

- Prepare and implement the yearly work plan as per the guidance from the IPC leader.
- Organize and conduct surveillance for HAIs and antimicrobial resistance.
- Investigate and address outbreaks and provide expert advice, analysis, and leadership in outbreak investigation and control.
- Oversee the implementation of and compliance with IPC practices.
- Assist the IPC committee in product and material evaluations.
- Control and audit methods of disinfection and sterilization and the effectiveness of systems developed to improve hospital cleanliness.
- Implement departmental training programs among HCWs.
- Support and participate in research and assessment programs at national and international levels.
- Participate in the development and operation of regional and national IPC initiatives.
- Participate in programs and initiatives to promote rational antimicrobial use.
- Ensure that patient care practices are appropriate to the level of patient risk.
- Participate in development and provision of teaching programs for the medical, nursing, and allied health staff, as well as all other categories of HCWs.

Surveillance of antibiotics resistant bacteria

The emergence and spreading of antibiotic resistant bacteria threatens treatment of bacterial infections and management of patients in hospitals [16]. In hospitals, especially ICUs were critically ill patients requiring multiple invasive procedures are admitted, the risk of acquiring opportunistic HCAIs is high. Consequently, acquisition of HCAIs with antibiotic resistant bacteria among critically ill or immunocompromised patients is increased morbidity and mortality mostly due to treatment failure.

For surveillance (explained in more detail in the next paragraph) of antibiotic resistance, bacteriology laboratory is the key partner in surveillance of antibiotics resistance (ABR) which aims in tracking of changes in bacteria populations, early detection of resistant strains of bacteria and supporting outbreaks investigations [16]. The essential core data generated in the laboratories for routine culture and susceptibility testing are stored in laboratory information systems can be accessed, collected and analysed to generate passive surveillance findings (report) on the increasing or decreasing trends of antibiotic resistance over a specified periodic time [16]. However, bacteriology laboratory can be used for active surveillance during or after hospital outbreak. Moreover, findings of antibiotics resistance patterns from surveillance can be used to generate local empirical treatment guidelines for initiation of effective antibiotic treatment of critically ill patients in ICUs while further laboratory reports awaiting.

Limitation of clinical bacteriology laboratory in clinical ABR surveillance is that, determination of antibiotic resistant infections in hospitals are caused by spreading of resistant bacteria or horizontal transfer of mobile genetic elements harboring resistant genes is not routinely done [17]. Also, clinical surveillance using clinical samples are not so much useful as in early warning of emerging pathogens and mechanisms of antibiotics resistance. Therefore, this calls upon bacteriologists from different discipline to strongly implement integrated surveillance system referring to the collaborative efforts of the "One Health" concept due to the complex epidemiology of ABR [18]. There is no barrier to the spreading of ABR bacteria existing in animals, food industry and environment to humans and causing infections of serious sequelae (i.e., death) [18]. Hence, bacteriology laboratory has a wide utility in early detection of emerging ABR bacteria and mechanisms of ABR from animals, food and environment to human medicine for effective IPC measures.

Surveillance

Surveillance (public health or hospital setting) is defined as the ongoing, systematic collection, analysis, and interpretation of health data, essential to the planning, implementation, and evaluation of public health practice, closely integrated with the timely dissemination to those who need to know [1]. Surveillance provides the descriptive epidemiological information; demographics which is age and sex (person information); where (place information); and dates, hours, days, months and years (timely or periodic information). For a surveillance to be ideal, it should accommodate the following factors; simple, sensitive, timely, acceptable, strong predictive value, representative, flexible and cost-effective. Also, surveillance define a problem, determine where an illness is occurring geographically, estimate the size of a health problem, portray the natural history of a disease, generate hypotheses in research, monitor changes in infectious agents, detect changes in health practices and facilitate emergency planning. For policy makers and stakeholders to act effectively and appropriately, they requires competent professionals to communicate scientific surveillance results as simple information and they should be part of planning, implementation and intervention. The major aim of effective surveillance is to produce valid scientific data and convert them into the useful information which may be used to initiate appropriate interventions. Because the aim of surveillance is to collect, analyze and utilize (in terms of dissemination) data so that a certain disease is put under control. If no intervention is planned, there is no need of wasting resources in collecting and analyzing data. To estimate the size of an outbreak and monitoring of the process and effectiveness of interventions, policy makers and stakeholders use a measurable factor known as indicators. This may be numbers of new cases of diarrhea in a community or number of confirmed cases of a disease in a hospital ward or unit.

Basically there are three major types of surveillance, namely; active, passive and syndromic [1]. *Active surveillance:* local or national health system employing staff members to initiate actively collect of information about health conditions health laboratories, medical clinics, healthcare providers and population in general. Though it is too expensive, active surveillance provides the complete, accurate and timely information. *Passive surveillance:* local or national health system receives alerting reports submitted from clinics, hospitals, or public health units. Passive surveillance information is difficult to control in terms of quality and timeliness however it is relatively inexpensive strategy which covers large areas for critical information for monitoring health outcomes in the communities and hospitals. **Syndromic surveillance:** it can be conducted actively or passively in which health system uses case definitions based entirely on clinical features without any clinical or laboratory confirmation of a disease for example collecting cases of "rash illness" as measles. This type of surveillance is inexpensive and faster but it is not specific because other syndromes are cutting across different diseases (e.g., rashes may be due to minor rubella infections) and one syndrome may mask the other (e.g., diarrhea due to rotavirus versus diarrhea due to cholera). Also, when a surveillance being active or passive but focuses in one disease for example Tuberculosis program or HIV program it is known as **categorical surveillance**. When a combination of passive and active surveillance investigates multiple diseases under the same infrastructure it is known as **integrated surveillance**. Sometime, health system may actively and repeatedly surveys risk behaviors known to cause a disease for example unprotected sex or alcoholism, this is termed as **behavior risk factor surveillance system (BRFSS)** [1].

Infectious disease outbreaks in hospitals

Infectious disease outbreak can be defined as a significant increase of the incidence rate of certain infectious disease in the community (public health) or hospital (hospital outbreak) above background level [19, 20]. For the responsible authorities to declare an outbreak in the community or hospital setting there should be at least two or more similar cases in the same defined time, place and other related factors such as age, sex, mode or route of transmission and exposures of the disease. To improve public health, health systems should strongly deal with all things that can pose threats to public health range from chronic illnesses (e.g., heart disease, diabetes, or cancers), environmental disasters (e.g., tornadoes, hurricanes, or earthquakes), biologic or chemical terrorism to infectious disease outbreaks (e.g., Ebola viruses, cholera, or influenza). A threat to public health can be detected or alerted from hospital records (e.g., birth records or infectious diseases outbreaks), surveys (e.g., schools or insurance companies), environmental monitoring systems, animal health records or voluntary individual person reporting. On the other hand, in the hospital (infectious disease outbreak) it should be the same case in the same ward or unit within 48 hours which is clinically diagnosed or laboratory confirmed [21]. Most of infectious diseases outbreaks (> 50%) in hospitals happen in the intensive care units where highly vulnerable patients are admitted hence increasing morbidity and mortality rates [21]. Therefore, whenever there is an alert of any infectious disease outbreak in the community or hospital setting, a team of medical professionals (e.g., doctors, nurses, and bacteriologists), epidemiologists, emergency responders, public health professionals and policy makers should acts accordingly as soon as possible. The aim is to treat those who are already infected and second to investigate the implicating causative agent, source of infection and cut-off all possible routes of spreading to put the disease under control and prevent further transmissions.

Types of infectious disease outbreaks in hospitals

Outbreaks are categorized depending on the way causative bacteria is contacted or spreading from one patient to another in the ward (or unit). There are three types of outbreaks namely point source outbreaks, continuing common source outbreaks and propagated outbreaks.

Point source outbreaks: the implicating bacteria located at a single point are infecting patients in a very short periodic time. For example, surface colonized patient with methicillin resistant Staphylococcus aureus (MRSA) in the same unit might be shading off this pathogen and resulting to an outbreak of hospital acquired-MRSA infections. This type of outbreak shows a bell-shaped epidemic curve, which is increasing very sharp to reach a peak and then decreasing very sharp.

Continuing common source outbreak: almost all cases are infected from the same source with the same causative bacteria over a very long period of time. For example, multidrug resistant Acinetobacter baumannii (MDR-A. baumannii) contaminating air conditioning machine (ventilator) may be circulating for a long period and responsible for hospital acquired pneumonia in ICUs until the source is identified and proper and effective measures are taken. In this kind of outbreak, epidemic curve does not increase sharply but reaches a plateau which exists for a long period until the source is identified and removed.

Propagated outbreaks: the causative agent is transmitted from one patient to another via certain vehicle or vector. In hospitals the common vehicle of transmission is contaminated hands of healthcare workers (HCWs). It may start as point source outbreak, but it can become a propagated outbreak. Through contaminated hands of HCWs, implicating pathogen is transmitted from source to contaminate other inanimate surfaces and medical instruments. Therefore patients are acquiring infection from either contaminated hands of HCWs, their immediate contaminated surfaces (e.g., beds or side tables) or medical supporting instruments (e.g., infusions' stand). Epidemic curve of this type of outbreak may show sharp increase but with incremental jumps indicating cases generation over specific time.

In hospitals, most of infectious disease outbreaks are due to cross-transmission of infectious agents between patients, or patients and healthcare workers or patients and environment. Similar cases in the same ward or unit, similar cases among similar patients, similar cases in the same short time interval and/or similar cases among healthcare workers and patients are clusters defining cross transmission of infection in hospital setting.

Bacteriologists are important members of the outbreak response team (ORT). They play a role in isolation of the pathogen responsible for outbreak, confirmation of suspected cases and processing and analyzing other non-biological specimens for investigating possible sources of outbreak for timely and effective control of the spreading routes hence putting the disease under control. With these key roles of bacteriologists in the investigation of an outbreak, definitely Bacteriology laboratory is also the most important investigation of an outbreak not only in hospitals but also in communities.

Epidemiologic steps to investigate an outbreak in a hospital setting

The decisions whether not to or to (and how extensively) investigate an outbreak depend on various factors including health related problems, department related factors and external concerns related factors. Health related problems such as source, mode or route of transmission, number of cases, severity of the illness, and the availability of effective prevention and control measures are considered before initiation of an investigation. Health departments consider to investigate an outbreak when the number of affected (or cases) patients is large than the background, when the disease is severe with high risk of complications, or death, effective control measures are available, and the potential of an outbreak to affect more other patients in ward or unit. For example, just one case of botulism is supposed to be investigated immediately because it is both potentially fatal and preventable. Therefore identifying and eliminating of the source is the main objective of an investigation. However, justification of most investigations is affected by either of the following: control or prevention of the health problem; research opportunity; public, political and legal issues; health program considerations; and opportunities of further training [22].

Before declaring existence of an outbreak and starting an investigation, it is important to be sure that an incidence of such a disease or infection is above the background level [23]. Then, epidemiologists and other professions should plan as soon as possible to start a "quick and clean" investigation [24]. Therefore, it is useful to have a systematic epidemiological approach to follow just to be sure that nothing is being missed. But before starting an investigation, there are four important questions epidemiologists and other professions should get answers from epidemiological approach they are setting. These questions are; what is the disease? What is the source? How is the disease being spread? How can the outbreak be stopped? [23].

Systematic epidemiological approach to follow during an outbreak in a hospital includes these steps;

1. Confirm the existence of an outbreak
2. Plan and prepare for the outbreak investigation
3. Construct a working case definition
4. Find cases systematically and record information
5. Perform descriptive epidemiology
6. Develop hypotheses
7. Evaluate hypotheses epidemiologically
8. As necessary, reconsider, refine, and re-evaluate hypotheses
9. Compare and reconcile with laboratory and/or environmental studies
10. Implement control and prevention measures
11. Initiate or maintain surveillance
12. Communicate findings

Confirm the existence of an outbreak

In a hospital ward or unit, an outbreak is the increased incidences of a disease cases than expected among over a particular defined period of time [20]. Most of the time, cases have common causative agent, mode or route of transmission, lists of exposure risks and similar clinical presentations. Some turns out to be true outbreaks of the same cause, others are sporadic with uncommon cases of the same disease and some are unrelated similar cases of unrelated diseases [22]. To verify that a cluster of cases is indeed an outbreak, the number of observed cases is compared with the number of expected cases. The expected number of cases is usually the number from the previous history over few weeks, months, or years [22].

Plan and prepare for the outbreak investigation

After confirming the existence of an outbreak in a hospital ward or unit, next step is to plan for conducting an investigation. The team should act very quickly while focusing to investigation's priorities and direction [23]. Investigation of an outbreak in a hospital requires a wide range of knowledge and skills therefore it is multidisplinary task, therefore a team of different professions known as outbreak response team (ORT) should be initiate [23]. ORT members should include; bacteriologists, clinicians, epidemiologists, environment health specialist, policy makers and stakeholders. Each member in the team has defined role and known reporting lines. Also, there supposed to be effective communication throughout an investigation. Moreover, first steps in identifying cases id directed to other hospital's wards or units and diagnostic bacteriology laboratory to conduct passive surveillance asking for previous reports of similar cases or active surveillance to initiate an investigation and collect additional information on new cases to be identified [22].

Bacteriology laboratory should be contacted for preparation of necessary resources required for appropriate specimen collections, transportations, and timely processing and reporting. Also, for record keeping of any laboratory reports produced. For bacterial outbreaks, it is important to collect other non-biological specimens such as environmental contaminations (i.e., patient's beds, water, ventilators and invasive devices) so as to investigate possible sources of an outbreak.

Construction of a working case definition

A case definition is a standard set of criteria for deciding whether a patient should be categorized as having the health condition of interest, this includes clinical criteria particularly in the setting where investigation of the outbreak is been conducted of which time, place, person are strictly considered. Such clinical criteria may include; fever > 40^0C, $\geq$ three loose bowel movement per day, convulsion or poor feeding among neonates. A tool used to classify if a patient is having or not having a disease of interest is known as case definition, although most of case definition are not 100% accurate in their classifications because some people with similar but not same illness/clinical criteria may be included and some people without or with mild symptoms may be missed [22]. For this reason a case definition may include, symptoms; laboratory results – for example isolation of implicating bacteria or its toxin, if it is known; when the illness occurred; where the illness occurred, for example specific ward or unit (e.g., neonatal ICU); patients' personal characteristics, such as age or sex; and different levels of uncertainty (confirmed cases – patient with positive laboratory result; probable cases – patient with typical symptoms of the illness but no laboratory confirmation; and possible cases – patient with fewer symptoms or unusual symptoms) [23].

Basically epidemiologists struggles to ensure the case definition includes almost all actually cases but also very few or no false positive cases included. However it is not always the case, because patients with no or having mild symptoms they will be missed for they have no reasons to be included in the investigation. Therefore, they definitely will be excluded from investigation [22].

Hypotheses development

Depending on the outbreak, this step involves interviewing patients identified as cases to gather information that may address the possible source of the agent, the mode of transmission (vehicle or vector) and the exposures of the disease [22, 23].

If the disease is known, it is better to be familiar with it by asking the following questions: What is the agent's usual reservoir? How it is usually transmitted? What vehicles are commonly implicated? What are the known risk factors? This at the very least will help in proposing and initiation of possible preventive and control measures while further investigation procedures are going on [22].

Epidemiological testing of hypotheses developed

At this step, hypotheses are tested to check if the source, mode of transmission and exposures of the disease were correctly identified. In the field, hypotheses are evaluated by examining the combination of environmental evidence, laboratory science, and epidemiology [24].

Laboratory science involves consultation of bacteriologists (they may be part of the ORT) and bacteriology laboratory for processing of clinical (human's) and environmental (environment) specimens [23]. Environmental specimens are part of investigation for the purpose of determining possible source of an outbreak which can be contaminated inanimate surfaces or source of water in the wards or unit. Therefore, core functions of bacteriology laboratory are diagnosis and confirmation of cases, records keeping and confirmation of sources of outbreaks for effective control measures (discussed later).

From epidemiological perspectives, two ways can be used to evaluate hypotheses; comparison between hypotheses and established facts or analytical epidemiology by quantifying relationships and examining the role of chance. Hypotheses are compared with established facts when hypotheses are obviously supported by clinical, laboratory, environmental and epidemiologic evidence [24].

Main areas where environmental evidence can be gathered are from analytical studies (cohort and case-control studies) and clinical and environmental investigation. Clinical and environmental investigation are carried out at the same time [23]. While diagnosing (confirming) cases, environment is also investigated as being potential source of outbreak i.e., contaminated inanimate hospital surfaces such as patient's beds and washing sinks (source of skin and soft tissue infections) and ventilators (source of hospital acquired pneumonia).

Identifying the original source of an outbreak

To identify the possible original source of outbreak in hospital ward or unit, environmental and colonization samples are mandatory. Environmental samples include water, medical instrument and immediate inanimate surfaces to the patients such as beds and side tables. Colonization specimens such as patients' rectal and nares swabs should be collected. On the other hand, healthcare workers' hands swab specimens may be part of an investigation. Most of outbreaks in hospitals occur due to cross-transmission between colonized or infected patients; patients and colonized or infected HCWs; and patients and contaminated inanimate surfaces.

Isolation of the same bacteria from clinical (e.g., blood, urine or wound swabs) and colonization (nares or rectal swabs) or environmental (patients' beds or side tables) or medical instrument (intubator or dialysis) specimens, preliminarily suggests possible cross-transmission hence potential source of an outbreak in the ward or unit. But, further analysis should be done to come out with conclusive report. This analysis include as simple as phenotypic antibiotic resistance profiling to as advanced as molecular techniques such as genotypic antibiotic resistance profiling and bacteria genomic profiling.

Phenotypic antibiotic resistance profiling: This technique compares antibiotic susceptibility patterns of two or more similar strains of bacteria from different sources (e.g., clinical or colonization or contamination) to establish possible preliminary source of an outbreak in the hospital [25, 26]. For example, two *Acinetobacter baumannii* resistant to all antibiotics except colistin, one is isolated from patient's blood sample and the other is isolated from swab of an infusion stand of the same patient, then the two bacteria are more likely to belong in the same clone. Therefore, contaminated infusion stand maybe potential source of this outbreak [27].

Similar patterns of drug resistance genes harbored by bacteria of different sources: Bacteria of different sources are compared by the presence of similar patterns of genes (e.g., extended spectrum beta-lactamases (ESBLs) i.e., *bla*OXA, *bla*IPM, *bla*KPC, *bla*TEM, *bla*SHV and *bla*CTX-M) conferring resistance to antibiotics. For example, K. pneumoniae isolated from two different sources, such as clinical and environment isolates, having the same patterns of ESBL genes, for example both isolates harboring *bla*CTX-M-15 and *bla*TEM-1 only, are considered similar. When they harbor different ESBL genes, one is harboring *bla*CTX-M-15 and *bla*TEM-1 while the other is harboring only one gene, either *bla*CTX-M-15 or *bla*TEM-1, the two bacteria are considered not similar [25].

Pulsed-field gel electrophoresis (PFGE): It is cost effective and gold standard technique in fingerprinting or genotyping of microorganisms. This technique involves digestion of core genomes of bacteria into deoxyribonucleic acid (DNA) fragments by restriction endonuclease enzymes such as *Asc*I, *Xba*I and *Apa*I. DNA fragments are then separated by gel electrophoresis according to their molecular weight by electric field in an alternating direction and a varying duration. First current of electric field moves from top to bottom at the central axis while the other two currents moving at an angle of 60 degrees each sides of the gel. On gel electrophoresis, two or more bacteria from different sources showing similar patterns of DNA fragment bands are linked together and their percentage of relatedness is calculated using different available software [28].

Multi locus sequence typing (MLST): It is DNA sequence based technique which is none time consuming. Bacteria species are characterized from internal fragment sequences of several (mostly, seven) housekeeping genes; *arc*C, *aro*E, *glp*F, *gmk, pta, tpi* and *yqi*L. In each housekeeping gene, distinct alleles are contained in specific loci called sequence type (ST). Genetic sequences are amplified and detected then matched between bacterial species if they originate from the same or different sequence types (ST) [29].

Whole genome sequencing (WGS): Complete sequencing of the chromosomal DNA of an organism to determine the likelihood and genetic relationships of DNA materials and susceptibility of diseases to specific source of an outbreak. It is direct DNA sequencing based technique which matches bacteria species at their genomic sequence level. This technique has high resolution above all the mentioned techniques because base by base of the bacteria genomes are sequenced and compared. It can detect even point of mutations that unable to change expression of proteins hence can detect the very small differences between bacterial strains [30, 31].

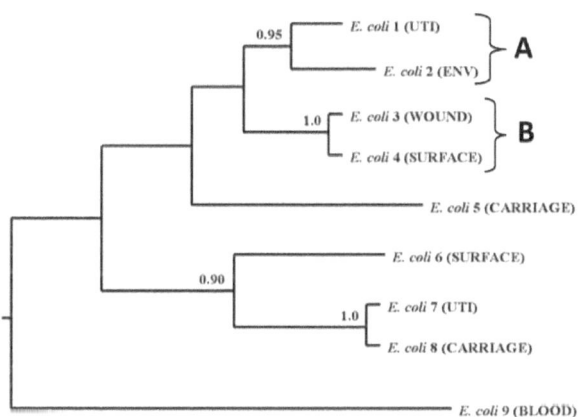

Figure 2: Illustration of a phylogenetic tree showing maximum likelihood of *E. coli* isolated from different sources. For example, (A). *E. coli* 1 isolated from urine (UTI) is genetically

resembling *E. coli* 2 isolated from environment (ENV) by 0.95 (95%). (B). *E. coli* 3 isolated from wound is genetically resembling *E.coli* 4 isolated from surface by 1.0 (100%). Therefore, it can be concluded that, contaminated inanimate surfaces (e.g., patient's bed) is the potential source of surgical site infections outbreak in a particular unit.

Controlling the outbreak

The major goals of an outbreak investigation are preventing further spreading of implicating bacteria and preventing future alike outbreaks. To achieve these major two goals, investigation team focuses on controlling the source, controlling of transmission or spreading route, and temporarily closing of the unit if the first two are not feasible.

Controlling the source: at this point, team focuses on the possible sources: colonization and inanimate contamination. If the source of an outbreak is a colonized patient(s), then isolation of specific patient(s) into a single room is an appropriate measure to prevent further shading off and transmission to other patients. But, observation and adhering to contact precautions is strictly recommended. However, contaminated inanimate surfaces or medical instruments can be potential source of an outbreak in a hospital. If this is the case, then major and effective decontamination and disinfection practices are therefore highly recommended.

Controlling transmission: here the team focuses in cutting all routes of transmission from original source to patients even if sources remain unknown. The routes of transmission can be a vector (e.g., other organism) or a vehicle (e.g., contaminated hands of HCWs). This is done when it takes too long to identify and control the source of an outbreak. Efforts may include isolation of colonized patient(s) into quarantined room and put restrictions of access. Sometimes, HCWs' hands play the role as vehicles for transmission of implicating bacteria from contaminated surfaces to patients and between patients. Therefore, effective hand hygiene practices among HCWs are highly recommended.

When to decide an outbreak is over

To be sure an outbreak is over, is when the incidence (prevalence) drops to normal (expected) number, called the background rate. From here, surveillance takes off to make sure no subsequent increase of cases above background rate. Then, debriefing meeting is called to evaluate effectiveness of control measures, if there is a need of further scientific studies, if there is a need of any improvement of surveillance or control measures and presence of any factor which hindered or compromised investigation. Also, the team discusses any possible solution(s) to factor(s) that compromised investigation.

Planning for more scientific studies

If further scientific studies like molecular epidemiological studies are needed, they are initiated at this step. Also, new-emerging pathogens need more studies to examine its natural habitat, diagnostic techniques, virulence factors and pathogenesis. Also, local treatment guideline can be established.

Communicate the findings of an outbreak investigation

Findings from outbreak should be communicated to all team members and other important partners. Communication is made in two forms; oral and written. Oral briefing of investigation findings to hospital management and local health authorities. Written report is submitted to local, national and when necessary to other higher authorities such as WHO or CDC. Final report comprises the characteristics of an outbreak, weakness of the infection prevention and control that contributed to an outbreak and interventions taken and their effectiveness.

References

1. Ali S, Birhane M, Bekele S, Kibru G, Teshager L, Yilma Y, Ahmed Y, Fentahun N, Assefa H, Gashaw M: **Healthcare associated infection and its risk factors among patients admitted to a tertiary hospital in Ethiopia: longitudinal study**. *Antimicrobial Resistance & Infection Control* 2018, **7**(1):2.
2. Agency PH: **What are healthcare associated infections (HCAIs)?** In.
3. WHO: **Report on the Burden of Endemic Health Care-Associated Infection Worldwide**. In.; 2011.
4. Ylipalosaari P, Ala-Kokko TI, Laurila J, Ohtonen P, Syrjälä H: **Intensive care acquired infection is an independent risk factor for hospital mortality: a prospective cohort study**. *Critical Care* 2006, **10**(2):R66.
5. Wang M, Wei H, Zhao Y, Shang L, Di L, Lyu C, Liu J: **Analysis of multidrug-resistant bacteria in 3223 patients with hospital-acquired infections (HAI) from a tertiary general hospital in China**. *Bosnian journal of basic medical sciences* 2019, **19**(1):86.
6. Landelle C, Pagani L, Harbarth S: **Is patient isolation the single most important measure to prevent the spread of multidrug-resistant pathogens?** *Virulence* 2013, **4**(2):163-171.
7. **Standard Precautions** [https://www.health.state.mn.us/facilities/patientsafety/infectioncontrol/pre/standard.html]
8. Sax H, Allegranzi B, Uckay I, Larson E, Boyce J, Pittet D: **'My five moments for hand hygiene': a user-centred design approach to understand, train, monitor and report hand hygiene**. *Journal of Hospital infection* 2007, **67**(1):9-21.
9. WHO: **Hand Hygiene When and How**. In.; 2009.
10. **The Northern Ireland regional infection prevention and control manual** [https://www.niinfectioncontrolmanual.net/standard-precautions]
11. Huang SS, Septimus E, Kleinman K, Moody J, Hickok J, Avery TR, Lankiewicz J, Gombosev A, Terpstra L, Hartford F: **Targeted versus universal decolonization to prevent ICU infection**. *New England Journal of Medicine* 2013, **368**(24):2255-2265.
12. **Safe injection practices** [https://www.premiersafetyinstitute.org/safety topics az/safe injection-practices/safe-injection-practices/]
13. Hayleeyesus SF, Cherinete W: **Healthcare waste generation and management in public healthcare facilities in Adama, Ethiopia**. *Journal of Health and Pollution* 2016, **6**(10):64-73.
14. Organization WH: **Safe health-care waste management: policy paper**. In: *Safe health-care waste management: policy paper.* edn.; 2004.
15. Curless MS, Gerland CMA, Thompson CE: **Infection Prevention and Control**. 2018.
16. Johnson AP: **Surveillance of antibiotic resistance**. *Philosophical Transactions of the Royal Society B: Biological Sciences* 2015, **370**(1670):20140080.
17. Tacconelli E, Sifakis F, Harbarth S, Schrijver R, van Mourik M, Voss A, Sharland M, Rajendran NB, Rodríguez-Baño J, Bielicki J: **Surveillance for control of antimicrobial resistance**. *The Lancet Infectious Diseases* 2018, **18**(3).e99-e100.
18. Bordier M, Binot A, Pauchard Q, Nguyen DT, Trung TN, Fortané N, Goutard FL. **Antibiotic resistance in Vietnam: moving towards a One Health surveillance system**. *BMC public health* 2018, **18**(1):1136.
19. Nsubuga P, White ME, Thacker SB, Anderson MA, Blount SB, Broome CV, Chiller TM, Espitia V, Imtiaz R, Sosin D: **Public health surveillance: a tool for targeting and**

monitoring interventions. *Disease control priorities in developing countries* 2006, **2**:997-1018.

20. John M: **A dictionary of epidemiology**: Oxford University Press; 2001.
21. Gastmeier P, Stamm-Balderjahn S, Hansen S, Nitzschke-Tiemann F, Zuschneid I, Groneberg K, Rüden H: **How outbreaks can contribute to prevention of nosocomial infection: analysis of 1,022 outbreaks**. *Infection Control & Hospital Epidemiology* 2005, **26**(4):357-361.
22. Dicker RC, Coronado Ft, Koo D, Parrish RG: **Principles of epidemiology in public health practice; an introduction to applied epidemiology and biostatistics.** 2006.
23. Organization WH: **Strengthening surveillance of and response to foodborne diseases: a practical manual. Stage 2: strengthening indicator-based surveillance.** 2017.
24. Palmer S: **Epidemiology in search of infectious diseases: methods in outbreak investigation.** *Journal of epidemiology and community health* 1989, **43**(4):311.
25. Asir J, Nair S, Devi S, Prashanth K, Saranathan R, Kanungo R: **Simultaneous gut colonisation and infection by ESBL-producing Escherichia coli in hospitalised patients.** *The Australasian medical journal* 2015, **8**(6):200.
26. Foxman B, Zhang L, Koopman JS, Manning SD, Marrs CF: **Choosing an appropriate bacterial typing technique for epidemiologic studies.** *Epidemiologic perspectives & innovations* 2005, **2**(1):10.
27. Atik TK, Atik B, Kilinç O, Bektöre B, Duran H, Selek BM, Ceken N, Baylan O, Özyurt M: **Epidemiological evaluation of an Acinetobacter baumannii outbreak observed at an intensive care unit.** *Saudi medical journal* 2018, **39**(8):767.
28. Control CfD, Prevention: **Standard operating procedure for PulseNet PFGE of Listeria monocytogenes.** *Centers for Disease Control and Prevention, Atlanta, GA: http://www cdc gov/pulsenet/PDF/listeria-pfge-protocol-508c pdf* 2013.
29. Tan J, Langvik M, Yang A, Turner B, Rico A, Jankowski S, Theelen J, Pradhan A, Nutter R: **Fast, accurate, and automated workflow for multi locus sequence typing of Staphylococcus aureus.** *Clinical Microbiology & Infection* 2006, **12**.
30. **Whole Genome Sequencing (WGS)** [https://www.cdc.gov/pulsenet/pathogens/wgs.html]
31. Salipante SJ, SenGupta DJ, Cummings LA, Land TA, Hoogestraat DR, Cookson BT: **Application of whole-genome sequencing for bacterial strain typing in molecular epidemiology.** *Journal of clinical microbiology* 2015, **53**(4):1072-1079.